AUTHENTIC FRENCH FASHIONS OF THE TWENTIES

413 Costume Designs from "L'Art et la Mode"

Edited and with an Introduction by

JoAnne Olian

Curator, Costume Collection
Museum of the City of New York

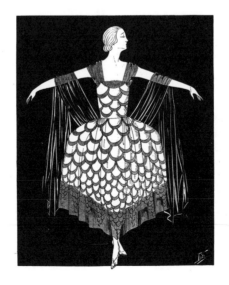

DOVER PUBLICATIONS, INC., NEW YORK

Copyright © 1990 by Dover Publications, Inc.
All rights reserved under Pan American and International Copyright Conventions.

Published in Canada by General Publishing Company, Ltd., 30 Lesmill Road, Don Mills, Toronto, Ontario.
Published in the United Kingdom by Constable and Company, Ltd., 10 Orange Street, London WC2H 7EG.

Authentic French Fashions of the Twenties: 413 Costume Designs from "L'Art et la Mode" is a new work, first published by Dover Publications, Inc., in 1990.

DOVER *Pictorial Archive* SERIES

Manufactured in the United States of America
Dover Publications, Inc., 31 East 2nd Street, Mineola, N.Y. 11501

Library of Congress Cataloging-in-Publication Data

Authentic French fashions of the twenties : 413 costume designs from
     "L'art et la mode" / edited by JoAnne Olian.
          p.   cm. — (Dover pictorial archive series)
     ISBN 0-486-26187-5
     1. Costume—France—History—20th century.   2. Art et la mode.
I. Olian, JoAnne.   II. Series.
GT880.A87   1990
391′.00944′09042—dc20   89-71440
                                              CIP

INTRODUCTION

The glossy fashion magazines of today trace their origins to the costume books of the sixteenth century, when voyages of exploration and discovery created an avid curiosity about the constantly widening world. So popular was the subject that these books were published all over Europe, but principally in Venice and Germany. The first such volume appeared in 1562 in Paris. Unlike modern publications, these books did not predict fashion, but depicted foreign dress and described the customs and manners of both the Old and the New World.

In the second half of the seventeenth century the focus shifted to France, where Jean-Baptiste Colbert, finance minister of Louis XIV, determined to build a strong economy, and, cognizant of the national predilection for fashion and luxury, based one aspect of this ambitious program on the manufacture of French textiles, instituting steep protective tariffs, prohibiting the wearing of foreign silks and establishing over 100 factories under crown patronage. The results of these measures were strikingly evident at the palace of Versailles, the showcase of the Sun King.

Court fashions appeared in *Le Mercure Galant*, but it was not until the last quarter of the eighteenth century, in response to the insatiable contemporary demand for novelty, that *Galerie des Modes* initiated new styles fresh from the dressmakers. Published from 1778 to 1787, it depicted the mercurial fashions of a society so obsessed with style and change that Abigail Adams, in a letter from Paris, wrote, "To be out of fashion is more criminal than to be seen in a state of nature—to which the Parisians are not averse."

In the nineteenth century, fashion periodicals, embraced by a growing middle class, proliferated rapidly. From 1840 to 1870 over 100 new magazines appeared in England, Germany and America as well as France. Adhering to a more or less uniform format, they covered social events, published new works of fiction and poetry, offered ideas for needlework projects and provided both color plates and black-and-white engravings of the latest fashions, which were invariably French.

The virtually simultaneous appearance on the fashion scene of Charles Frederick Worth and the Empress Eugénie assured permanent supremacy for French fashion. By her endorsement of Worth in the late 1850s, Eugénie was indirectly responsible for the creation of the haute-couture industry. Emperor Napoleon III, in the tradition of Louis XIV, limited the wearing of a gown at court to a single occasion, keeping mills and seamstresses busy producing a stream of novelties for a nouveau-riche society to wear to the palace of the Tuileries. As principal dressmaker to the glittering court of the Second Empire, Worth was responsible for the extravagant, hoop-skirted opulence of the Empress, who, by imperial command, dressed exclusively in Lyons silks. From 1867, when *Harper's Bazar* began publication, Worth became a household name in America, as he already was in France, through the fashion communiqués from Paris-based correspondent Emmeline Raymond. Success enabled Worth to transform the time-honored craft of the humble dressmaker, who merely executed gowns to a client's taste, into a major industry. At the House of Worth 1400 employees translated each new collection into custom-made gowns for its wealthy and titled international clientele. In the late nineteenth century, American importers were making seasonal buying trips to Paris on behalf of their customers. By 1924 exports of women's clothing worldwide amounted to 500 million francs.

The format established by Worth remains the method practiced by the French couture. Each year a house presents two collections of original models by its designer, which are shown on live mannequins at openings attended by the press, private clients and buyers for specialty shops abroad. Samples and models chosen by clients are custom made individually in the firm's atelier. This system was employed by designers such as Callot Sœurs, Cheruit, Doucet, Martial & Armand, Molyneux, Patou, Poiret and others whose designs appeared frequently in *L'Art et la Mode* to launch their collections at shows for a select invited audience. Magazines such as *L'Art et la Mode* were read avidly not only by the rich who patronized the couture, but also by the woman who relied on her "little dressmaker" to copy the styles depicted in the periodicals. This practice was widespread in Europe, where a woman who aspired to be well-dressed eschewed ready-made apparel until the 1950s, when *prêt-à-porter* became an accepted alternative to custom-made clothing.

In the 1920s, fashion magazines remained the principal source for news of the latest Paris gowns; *Vogue* and *Harper's Bazaar* continued to devote most of their fashion coverage to the French couture. *L'Art et la Mode*, sold on both sides of the Atlantic, provided bilingual captions as well as English synopses of its columnists' contributions. Enjoying remarkable longevity (1880 to 1967), it had the distinction of publishing the first halftone illustration ever printed in a fashion magazine. Appearing every Saturday, it managed to find sufficient style news to fill every issue. Twice a year the new collections were published, and two millinery issues also appeared annually. Garb worn at social events by well-known Parisiennes was described in detail, plays were discussed and opinions on manners, mores and fads were proffered by "Frivoline," while "Magda" covered style news. The fashion drawings are of several categories: dressmakers' advertisements, stage wardrobes (a favorite way for couturiers to expose their creations to the public), garments invented by *L'Art et la Mode*'s illustrators and the latest fashions credited to a designer or available in pattern form, portrayed in settings of the chic events and watering places frequented by the *haut monde*.

The fashionable Parisienne, following an undeviating annual schedule that resembled nothing so much as a royal progress, attended the Bal des Petits Lits Blancs (a children's benefit), went to the races at Auteuil and Longchamp and was seen at the opening of the Ballets Russes in June just before leaving for Deauville, "the smartest summer resort in Europe" according to *Vogue*, which enumerated its attributes including "above all gowns and gowns and gowns." September found *tout Paris* in Biarritz, then back to town after the hunting season for fashion shows, fittings, galas at the Cercle Interallié, subscription performances at the Opéra, theater and the Bal de la Couture sponsored by the Chambre Syndicale for the benefit of needy sewing workers, ending with Réveillon (Christmas Eve) suppers before beginning the annual round on the Côte d'Azur or St. Moritz.

L'Art et la Mode captures the glamour that was Paris in the twenties. Its pages evoke Art Deco, Sunday evening at the Ritz, the Casino de Paris, jazz at the Bœuf sur le Toit, the legendary Josephine Baker at the Folies-Bergère and Paul Poiret stepping off the Train Bleu at Cannes, where golf was de rigueur until 5 P.M. and the Casino the in spot until 5 A.M.

The streamlining of life dictated the streamlining of line, the hallmark of the decade. The contemporary aesthetic was manifested in the seemingly paradoxical union of utter simplicity of form with unlimited luxury of materials. Equally true in art, architecture, the decorative arts and fashion, this visual philosophy was epitomized in the Exposition Internationale des Arts Décoratifs et Industriels Modernes held in Paris in 1925 on the banks of the Seine, where the Pavillon de l'Elégance occupied a central position among the buildings of the fair.

Reverberations of this paring down were felt far beyond art and fashion. As the cocoon of layers of cloth was discarded, years were shed and restrictions carried over from the nineteenth century were rejected. Youth emerged from this chrysalis to find nothing too daring, too dangerous or too unusual as long as it was new. The boyish figure, actually more like that of a soignée adolescent, was the visual manifestation of this attitude. The adaptation of men's fashions for women enjoyed considerable popularity. Gabrielle Chanel wore a man's sweater on the Riviera, creating a new fashion. In 1925, *L'Art et la Mode* wrote, "In all the new collections an important place is reserved for the 'masculine' type of tailored suit. The coat is cut on the lines of a man's overcoat." Some women even had their clothing made by

men's tailors, and in chic circles it was considered amusing for a couple to appear together in "le smoking," masculine evening wear (p. 108). The fashion for the "tailleur strict," or man-tailored suit, emphasized the sharp demarcation between day and evening garb, and was embraced by the new woman who smoked in public, painted her lips and nails red and knew how to wield a cocktail shaker.

Above all, the twenties were young. The statuesque woman gave way to the asexual, lithe girl. The mysterious swathing and exotic draperies of prewar garments whose natural habitat was night, were suddenly passé. The splendor of Poiret looked old-fashioned next to the sportive look of Chanel and Patou, seen in its element out-of-doors.

Perhaps the most significant influence on fashion in the twenties was the growing popularity of sports among women. When Suzanne Lenglen appeared at Wimbledon in 1921 in a sleeveless sweater, a short pleated skirt by Patou and a yellow bandeau on her hair, she was the harbinger of a revolution. Even if one's most strenuous exercise was walking to the car, Patou's sportive look was rapidly pervading fashion. During the 1924 Olympics, *L'Art et la Mode* published an entire issue devoted solely to *élégances sportives*. While Chanel appealed to the rich woman who wanted to look understated and modern, Jean Patou, whose clientele was young and international, was considered by Poiret to be the greater threat. Asserting that the new woman appeared to be made of cardboard, Poiret expressed fear for the future of the couture. His voice was distinctly a minority one, as smart society flocked to the new Mediterranean resorts of St. Raphael and Menton, where they passed the time on the beach in pyjamas or bathing suits, acquiring a newly chic suntan as they anointed themselves with Patou's "Huile de Chaldée."

The automobile was the technological symbol of the twenties. To women, who had learned to drive ambulances and tractors during World War I, it represented the extension of their new-found freedom and status. By 1921 couturiers were even making a specialty of motoring apparel. This new mobility simplified the move from resort to resort, as Parisians motored down to Deauville, only 120 miles away, for the weekend, causing *L'Art et la Mode* to remark that Paris was fast becoming a town where "smart society women pass a few days in between seasons."

Equal in importance to sports and the automobile to an understanding of the radical change occurring in fashion, was the 1922 novel, *La Garçonne*, by Victor Margueritte, which caused such a scandal that its author was stripped of his Legion of Honor. The heroine, a student at the Sorbonne, embodied the movement toward sexual equality. Disillusioned by the hypocrisy of society, she broke with her parents and fiancé, cut her hair, wore men's clothing, became a successful businesswoman, smoked opium and had many love affairs, including a lesbian relationship. *La Garçonne* was the model for a generation that found its physical expression in flattened breasts and hips, short hair and short skirts that allowed freedom of movement without the anachronistic encumbrances of extraneous layers of cloth or restrictive corsets.

The style we think of as twenties did not emerge fully formed with the advent of the decade. The years 1920 through 1927 were marked by enormous changes, from the windblown naïveté of the early twenties to the androgynous, shingle-coiffed sophisticate of 1927. Stylistic changes can be clearly seen in the attitudes delineated in fashion illustrations. While the early figures seem at the mercy of each passing breeze, the later ones convey an air of assurance and ease. In much the same way, clothing exemplifies the change from fussy ruffles to controlled and defined pleats.

The sharp contrast between the fashions of 1920 and 1927 did not develop in an ordered sequence. Fashion emerged after World War I in a state of confusion. Some designers looked backward for inspiration, while others, sensitive to the changes in women's lives and requirements, searched for a new vocabulary, resulting in a cacophony of eclecticism that did not fuse into a harmonious style until almost the mid-twenties.

In 1920 hemlines were at mid-calf, and waistlines were normal. Skirts began to drop in 1921, dipping almost to the ankles by 1922, followed by the waistline, which settled on the hips. This attenuated silhouette was emphasized by vertical pleats and embroidered panels. The winter collections of 1923 marked the beginning of a slowly rising hemline that paused below the calf in fall 1924, a season also characterized by an increasing simplicity, accentuated by tailored belts with buckles. The trend toward shorter skirts continued until 1927 when they reached unprecedented heights—actually only to just below the knee in the most extreme cases. Some couturiers raised hems only to mid-calf and many dresses were longer in back or on the sides, a portent of longer skirts to come. Matching coat and dress ensembles were very fashionable. Skirts were flared, pleated and full of motion. The waistline was almost back to normal and bloused effects or draped panels created a new softness foreshadowing the clinging bias cut of the 1930s.

As clothing evolved, millinery and hairstyles followed. The wide skirts of the immediate postwar years were balanced by large hats that rested on long hair pulled back into a bun or knot. By 1922 the long, narrow silhouette demanded smaller brims requiring less hair, which, by 1924, was generally bobbed. As the cloche hat became smaller and deeper, the shingled coiffure, so much a part of the garçonne look, became a necessity. Even chic little girls had their hair cut in this fashion (p. 125).

While the dominant trend was the tailored look, minor chords were also sounded, seemingly in all the collections at the same time. A perennial favorite of many couturiers was the robe de style, a full-skirted dress with stiffened panniers in the manner of the eighteenth century or the crinoline of Eugénie. A Second Empire ball held in Paris in 1922 and an exhibition the following September in Biarritz helped to account for the continuing popularity of this romantic style. While the excesses of Poiret were démodé for daytime, the opulence of the East remained the inspiration for much of the evening fashion. Lamés and lavishly beaded metallic brocades were the guise under which the Orient flourished.

Simplification of cut gave rise to surface ornamentation in the form of fringe, beading or embroidery. Ethnic influences of all kinds were fashionable, especially the Romanian embroidered blouses so popular with women and their daughters. "Russian" collars and, most important, "Spanish" shawls were seen frequently in *L'Art et la Mode*, while the discovery of Tutankhamen's tomb in 1922 inspired the couture in new realms of exotica (p. 57).

F. Scott Fitzgerald remarked that "Part of the enchantment of Paris in the Twenties was that everything that happened there seemed to have something to do with art." The influence of Cubism on fashion is undeniable, both in the style of illustration and the clothes themselves. Flattened, impossibly elongated figures attest to Cubist influence as well as that of Marie Laurencin and Modigliani. The asymmetry, geometrically precise pleats and tubular forms of dresses and figures relate directly to painting.

Art and couture enjoyed a close relationship throughout this period. Poiret's sister, Nicole Groult, on intimate terms with the renowned painters of the day, was said by Picasso to capture the spirit of modern art in dress. Groult was a close friend of Laurencin, with whom she shared a palette of grayed pastels, emphasized by strokes of black. Poiret, whose wit and theatricality were natural attributes for the stage, designed numerous ballets and revues, notably *Vogue* in 1921, in which actors were artfully costumed as chess pieces, dominoes and Venetian glass. Chanel designed costumes inspired by Attic pottery for Cocteau's 1921 production of *Antigone*, for which Picasso painted sets and masks. If a single dramatic event could be said to encompass the aesthetic mood of the twenties, it might well be *Le Train Bleu*, which had its premiere at the Ballets Russes in 1924 during the Olympic games in Paris. It was set on the Riviera, and dancers costumed by Chanel portrayed bathers and golf champions, while the role of tennis star Suzanne Lenglen was danced by the ballet's choreographer, Bronislava Nijinska.

Textile design was intimately related to painting. Raoul Dufy designed silks and shawls for Bianchini (p. 58) and Sonia Delaunay created both Cubist clothing and fabrics, which were clearly the inspiration for many of the patterned materials of the decade.

Textiles with unusual names appear throughout *L'Art et la Mode*. They were short-lived novelty fabrics or names given by different mills to their version of a familiar material. The most popular cloth of the day was "Kasha," a fine, very soft twill flannel of vicuña or cashmere, developed by Rodier. Equally desirable were silk crepes of all weights, including *crêpe de chine*, *crêpe marocain* and *crêpe romain*. A flowery essay in *L'Art et la Mode*, defining history through textiles, selected Kasha and crepe as the quintessential fabrics of the twenties. Also fashionable were serge (often navy blue), Poiret twill, Duvetine (a coating fabric with a velvety nap) and jersey knitted of silk or wool. Printed silk foulards, voile and organdy were summer favorites. Linen did not make a postwar appearance until 1923 (perhaps, *Vogue* speculated, it had been needed in airplanes, and a flax crop takes seven years to reach maturity). With the exception of evening wear, the rich jewel colors of a decade earlier were replaced by black, white and Chanel's beloved beige.

Evening fabrics, often shot with metallic threads, were chiffon, sinuous silk velvets, lace and satin. Silver, seen in Poiret's chain-mail tunic (p. 42), was preferred to gold in lamé, embroidery and brocades. Platinum in combination with onyx or crystal, and pearls were much admired for jewelry and accessories. The fur coat was the height of fashion. Sable, mink, chinchilla and ermine were the ultimate luxury, but mole and red fox–trimmed leopard were considered high style. Fur trims, used lavishly, were monkey, squirrel, broadtail and skunk.

Leather, popular for outer wear, particularly for sportcoats and raincoats, also trimmed many tailored ensembles. An important innovation, seen on a leather raincoat of 1926 (p. 121), is the zipper shown here as a pocket closing.

Each couture house was known for its signature which attracted a particular type of client. Chanel and Patou appealed to the young moderns, in contrast to Worth, which specialized in wedding dresses and dignified elegance for the Old Guard. The robe de style was the forte of Jeanne Lanvin, who had made children's dresses before turning her hand to haute couture. Poiret toured the United States with a troupe of mannequins to show his dramatic evening clothes. Master of the grand gesture, he had three barges as his salon at the Art Deco exposition, while the Collectivité de la Couture was content to occupy the nearby Pavillon de l'Elégance. Madeleine Vionnet's "deceptively simple little things" were cut on the bias with such extraordinary skill that would-be imitators discovered they were "complex enough if one tried to copy them." Lucile and Boué Sœurs specialized in pastel taffetas iced with lace and rosettes of ribbon.

One of a new breed was Georges et Janin, which opened in 1923 and typified the smaller house making less-expensive gowns that still managed to bear the hallmark of the Parisian couture. Unique to Paris were maisons de couture devoted exclusively to children's clothes. Fairyland (p. 132) was one of three that operated in the same manner as the grand dressmaking establishments: Collections were presented every season at openings attended by a discriminating clientele of mothers and daughters from North and South America as well as France. *L'Art et la Mode* reflects a time when haute couture for children was as much a social statement as jeans and running shoes are in today's world.

Like all fashion magazines, *L'Art et la Mode* made a profound statement whose deceptively frivolous appearance belies its significance as cultural history. That line drawings of beaded dresses at Biarritz have been superseded by fashion photographs shot on location in corners of the world so remote they would have appeared only in *National Geographic* in the twenties only exemplifies the French adage, "The more things change, the more they remain the same," for, in a totally updated format, today's fashion magazine mirrors society no less accurately than the fashion magazine of the past reflected its world.

"Fashion . . . dies the minute it is born."—Gabrielle Chanel

JoAnne Olian
New York City
December 23, 1988

NOTE: Many of the captions in *L'Art et la Mode* appeared in French and English, in some instances the English being a condensed adaptation of the French. JoAnne Olian has corrected and expanded English captions where necessary, and has replaced the original French headings with new translations.

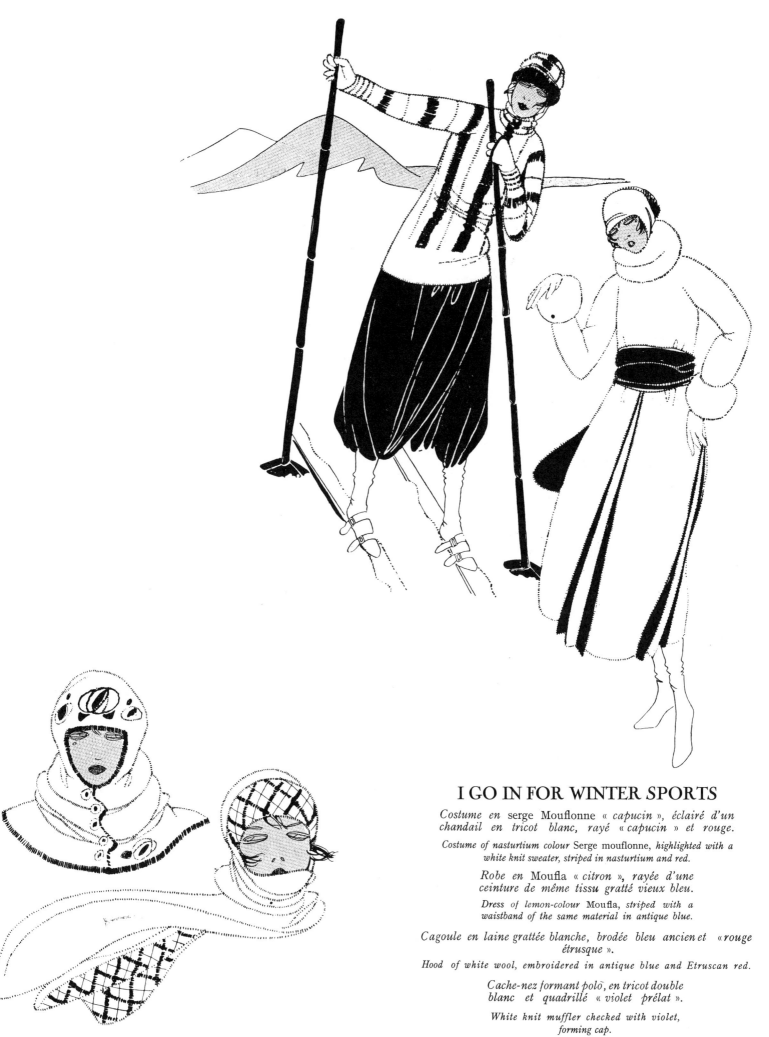

I GO IN FOR WINTER SPORTS

Costume en serge Mouflonne « capucin », éclairé d'un chandail en tricot blanc, rayé « capucin » et rouge.

Costume of nasturtium colour Serge mouflonne, highlighted with a white knit sweater, striped in nasturtium and red.

Robe en Moufla « citron », rayée d'une ceinture de même tissu gratté vieux bleu.

Dress of lemon-colour Moufla, striped with a waistband of the same material in antique blue.

Cagoule en laine grattée blanche, brodée bleu ancien et « rouge étrusque ».

Hood of white wool, embroidered in antique blue and Etruscan red.

Cache-nez formant polo, en tricot double blanc et quadrillé « violet prélat ».

White knit muffler checked with violet, forming cap.

Drawing by MEIGNOZ.

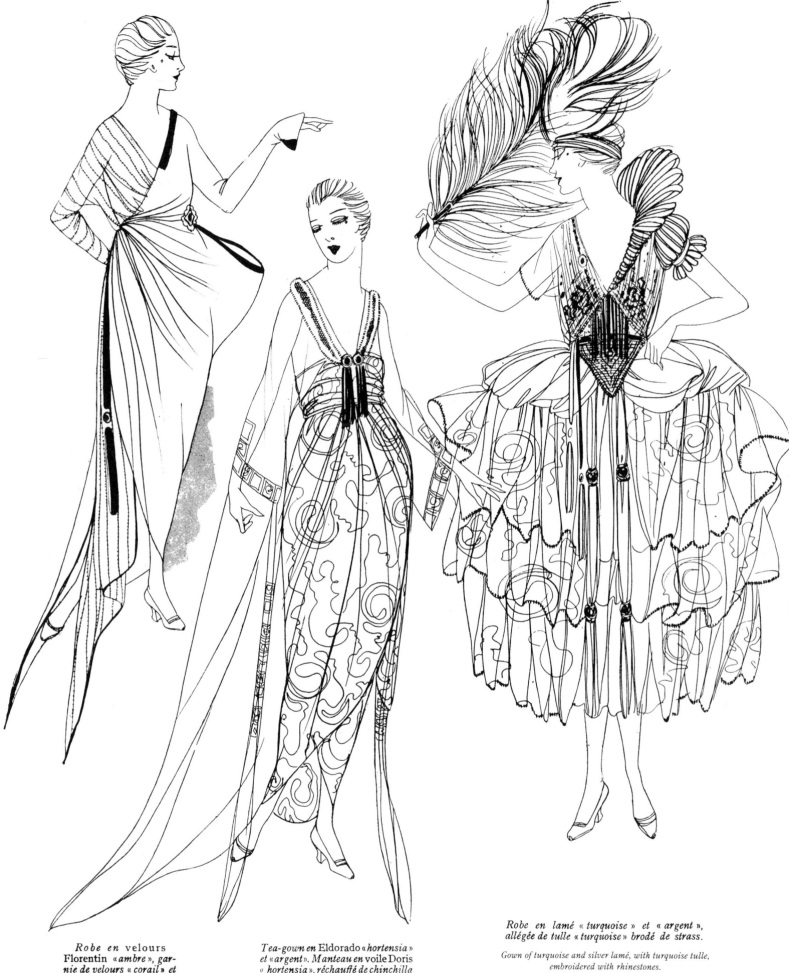

Robe en velours
Florentin *«ambre», gar-
nie de velours «corail» et
tulle gris, perlé de strass.*

Gown of amber colour Flo-
rence velvet, **trimmed with
coral colour velvet and grey**
tulle, with rhinestones.

Tea-gown en Eldorado *«hortensia»
et «argent». Manteau en* voile Doris
*« hortensia », réchauffé de chinchilla
et brodé d'argent.*

Tea-gown of hydrangea colour and silver
Eldorado. Mantle of hydrangea colour
Doris voile, with chinchilla, and embroi-
dered in silver.

*Robe en lamé « turquoise » et « argent »,
allégée de tulle « turquoise » brodé de strass.*

Gown of turquoise and silver lamé, with turquoise tulle,
embroidered with rhinestones.

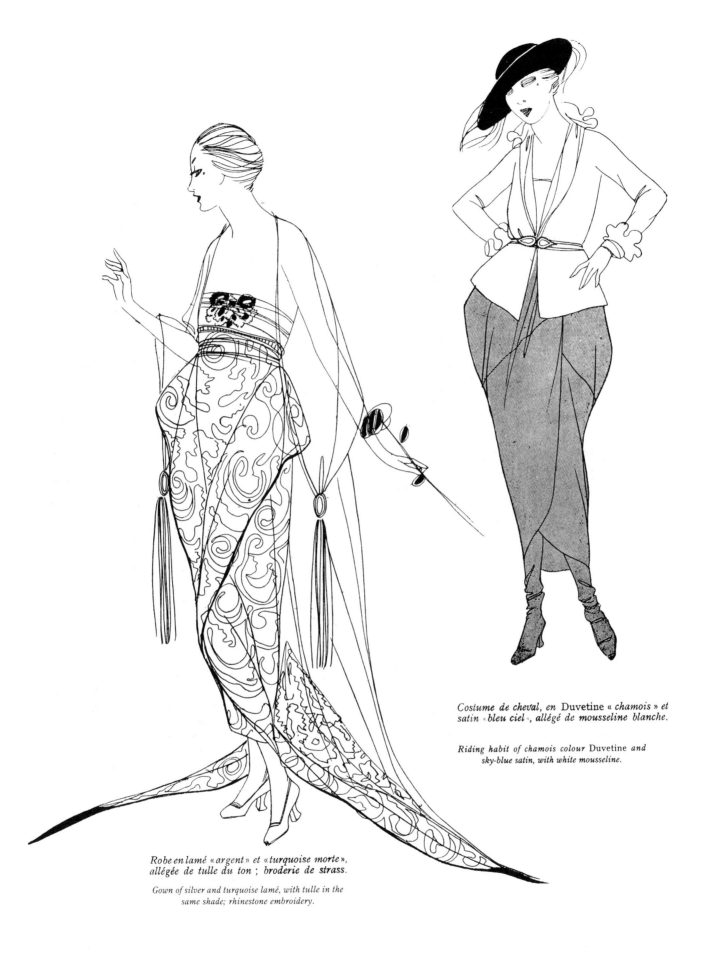

*Robe en lamé « argent » et « turquoise morte »,
allégée de tulle du ton ; broderie de strass.*

Gown of silver and turquoise lamé, with tulle in the
same shade; rhinestone embroidery.

*Costume de cheval, en Duvetine « chamois » et
satin « bleu ciel », allégé de mousseline blanche.*

Riding habit of chamois colour Duvetine and
sky-blue satin, with white mousseline.

THE ENSEMBLES WORN BY MADEMOISELLE CÉCILE SOREL

(REVIVAL OF *PRINCE D'AUREC* AT THE COMÉDIE-FRANÇAISE).

CREATIONS BY LUCILE

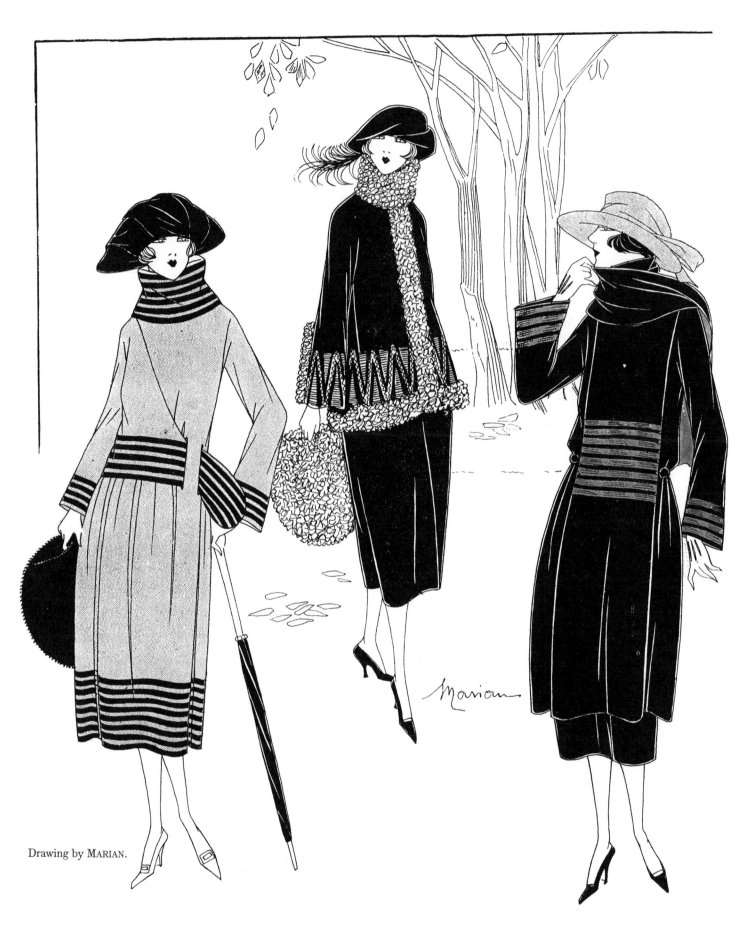

Drawing by MARIAN.

Robe en Sergella «*gris argent*», *garnie de petits galons cirés noirs.*

A dress made of silver grey Sergella, trimmed with shiny black, narrow braid.

Costume en Drapella *noir, orné* d'Agnella *et de broderie grise.*

Costume made of black Drapella, trimmed with Agnella and grey embroidery.

Costume en Velursine « *marine* », *orné de galons mohair.*

Costume made of navy Velursine, trimmed with mohair braid.

MORNING FANCIES

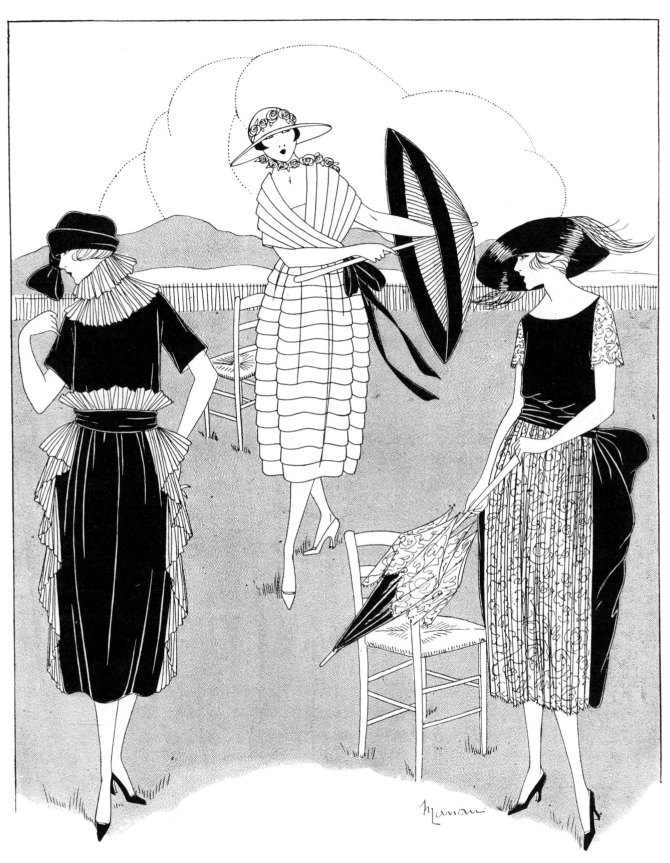

Drawing by MARIAN.

Robe de taffetas Libellule noir et voile plissé « citron ».

A dress made of black Libellule taffeta and lemon pleated voile.

Robe d'organdi « glycine », ceinture de velours noir.

A dress made of wisteria coloured organdy with a belt of black velvet.

Robe en Malines plissée et taffetas changeant rose et jaune.

A dress made of pleated Malines lace and changeablé pink and yellow coloured taffeta.

AT THE POLO CLUB

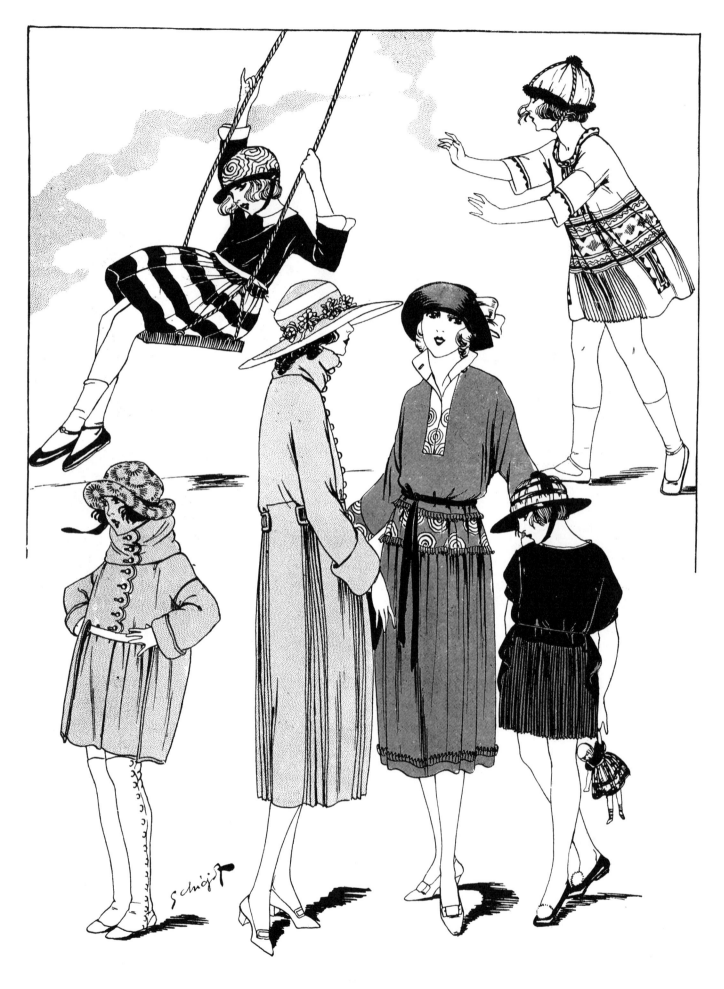

CHILDREN'S FASHIONS

Drawing by G. Chigot.

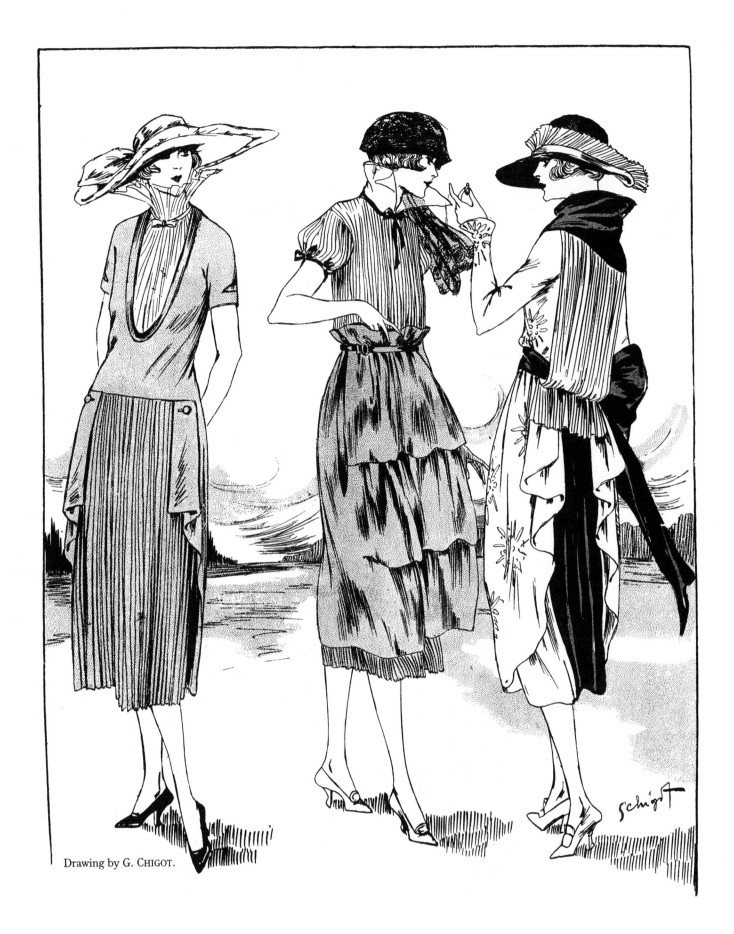

Drawing by G. CHIGOT.

Robe en shantung
«vert salade» et organdi.

A dress made of green shantung and organdy.

Robe en taffetas marine
et organdi blanc.

A dress made of navy blue
taffeta and white organdy.

Robe en satin tête de nègre
et organdi jaune, brodé jaune.

A dress made of brown satin and yellow organdy, embroidered in yellow.

SIMPLE DRESSES

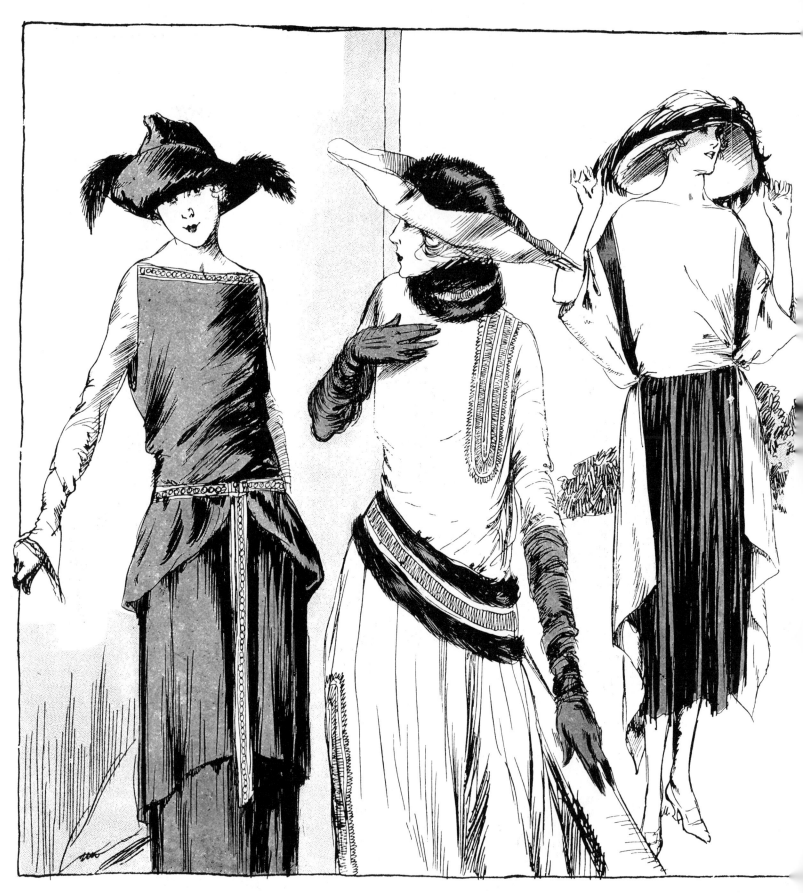

Tailles longues et tailles plus longues encore, mélange de Renaissance italienne et d'Hellénisme fantaisiste... Velours Salomé « châtaigne » et galons d'argent d'où s'échappent des manches de drap blanc.

A dress made of « chestnut » coloured Salomé velvet and silver braid. White wool sleeves.

Beaucoup de galons d'acier alternés de loutre rappelleront sur beaucoup de robes les ornements militaires des hussards, surtout sur celle-ci, faite de Drapella blanc.

A dress made of white Drapella, steel grey braid, otter fur bands.

La cape, transposée en dos de jaquette ou de corsage — crêpe Mireille blanc et mousseline « plomb » —, rendra libre la taille à la hauteur des reins. Ligne nouvelle que nous aimerons cet hiver.

A dress made of white Mireille crêpe and lead coloured mousseline.

THE SEASON

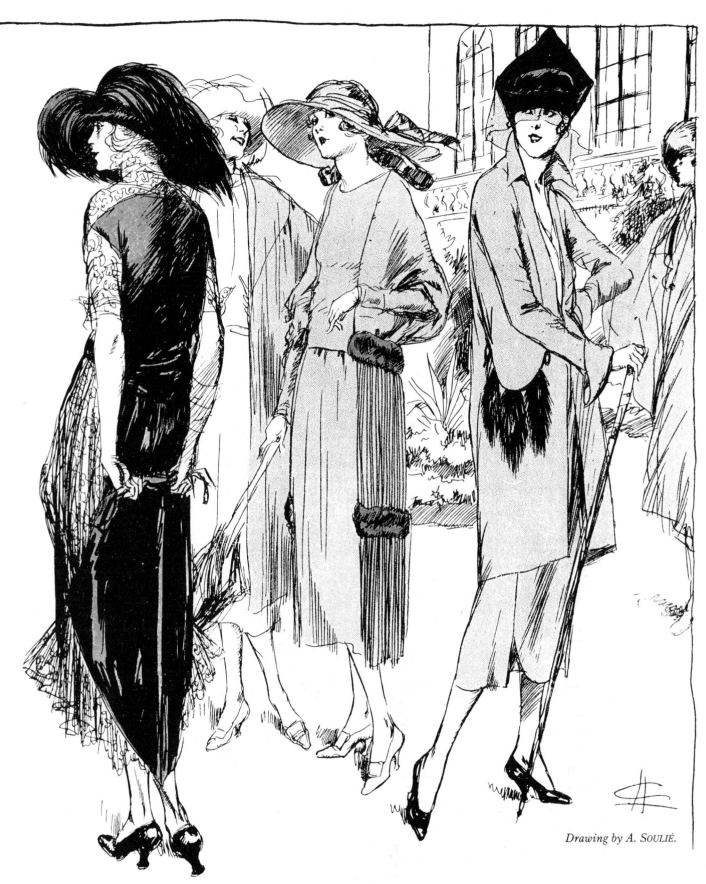

Drawing by A. SOULIÉ.

*La dentelle espa-
gnole revivra, mê-
lée à de la Fulgu-
rante noire.*

A dress made of black Fulgurante and Spanish lace.

*Ici encore, en Kasha «feuille
d'automne», nous retrouvons
ce mouvement de cape dra-
pée, soulignée de taupe.*

A dress made of « autumn leaves »
coloured Kasha and mole fur.

*Ne cherchez pas de ligne nouvelle dans
les «tailleurs»; seules, les garnitures les
renouvelleront ; ici, ce sont des queues
de skungs et son col montant.*

A suit trimmed
with skunk tails.

AT BIARRITZ

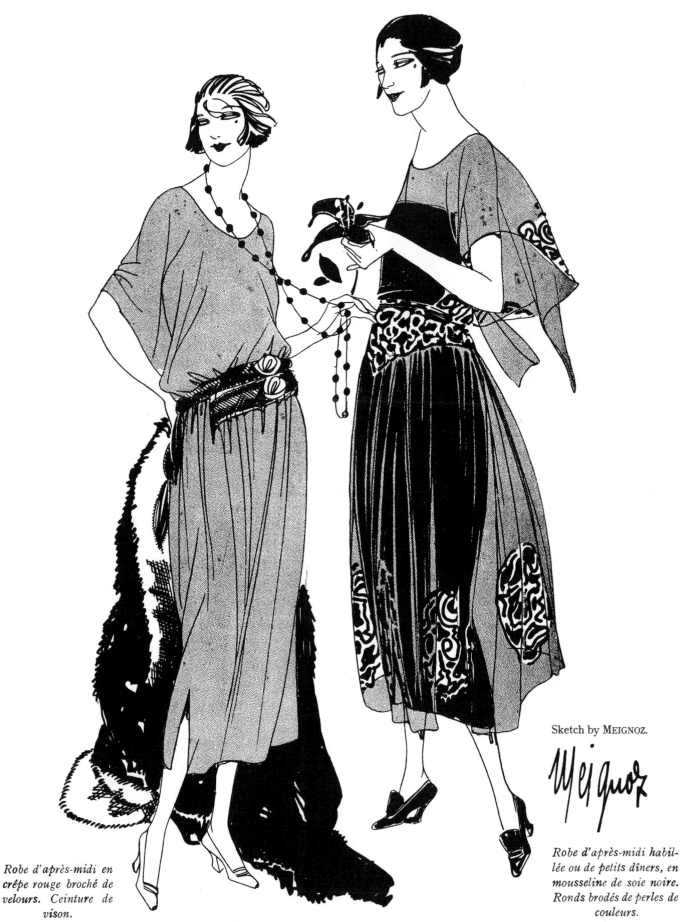

Sketch by MEIGNOZ.

Robe d'après-midi en crêpe rouge broché de velours. Ceinture de vison.

An afternoon gown made of red crêpe brocaded in velvet. Mink belt.

Robe d'après-midi habillée ou de petits dîners, en mousseline de soie noire. Ronds brodés de perles de couleurs.

An evening gown made of black chiffon, trimmed with coloured beads.

CREATIONS FROM PAQUIN

3, Rue de la Paix

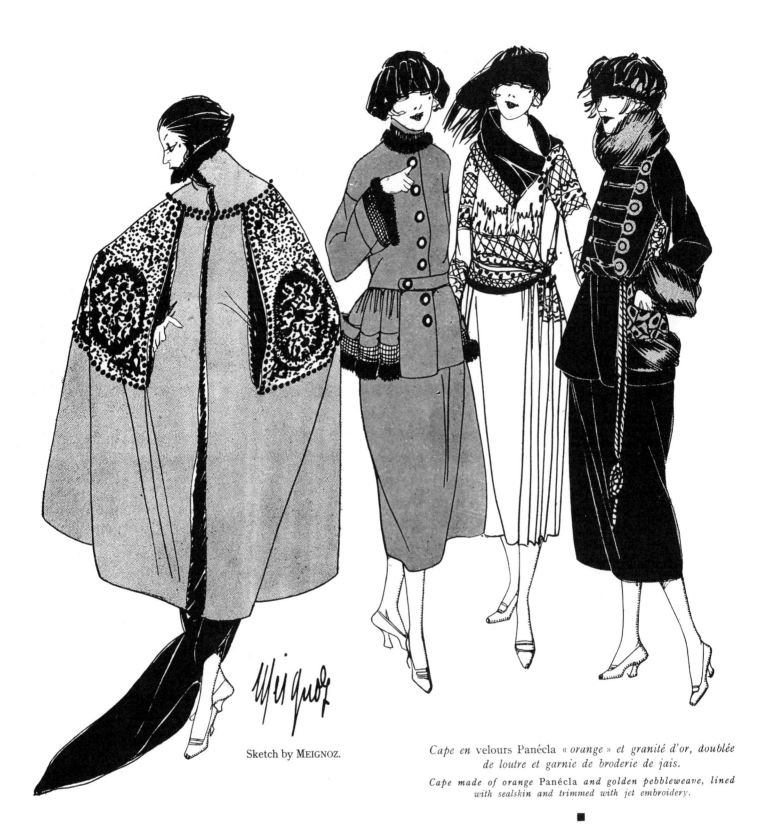

Sketch by MEIGNOZ.

CREATIONS
FROM
POIRET

Cape en velours Panécla « *orange* » *et granité d'or, doublée de loutre et garnie de broderie de jais.*

Cape made of orange Panécla *and golden pebbleweave, lined with sealskin and trimmed with jet embroidery.*

∎

Tailleur en Sergella « *marine* », *garni de galons rouges ourlés de peluche noire.*

Suit made of navy blue Sergella, *trimmed with red braid edged with black plush.*

∎

Robe en Kashavella « *gris ramier* » *à impressions marocaines noires, garnie de velours noir et fermée par un motif d'acier.*

A dress made of dove coloured Kashavella *with Moroccan designs, trimmed with black velvet and fastened with a steel ornament.*

∎

Tailleur en velours « *Corinthe* » *brodé de soie et d'applications grises. Renard gris.*

A suit made of plum coloured velvet embroidered with silk and appliquéd in grey fox.

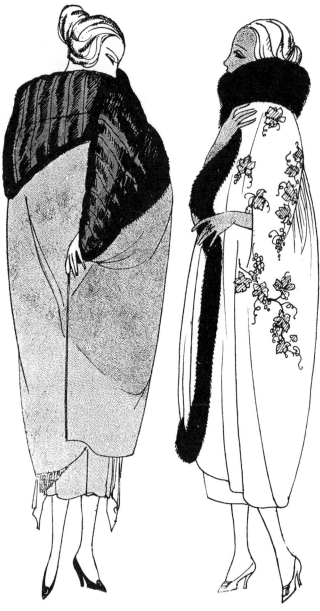

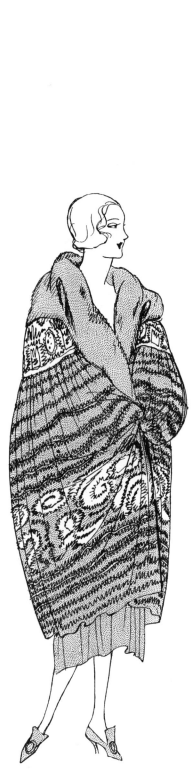

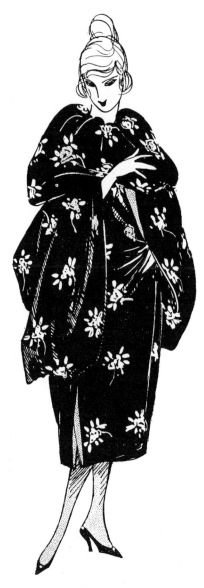

*Cape en crêpe de
'Chine « bleu-de-
roi », avec grand
col de kolinsky.*

*Royal blue crêpe
de chine cape
with large kolin-
sky collar.*

Gabrielle CHANEL

*Manteau de velours «vert lu-
mière», doublé de noir. Col et
garniture de renard noir. Broderie de pampres d'argent.*

*Green light velvet coat,
lined in black. Collar and
trim of black fox. Silver-
embroidered vine motif.*

PREMET

*Manteau froncé dans un
empièecement en tulle
Chantilly « taupe », re-
brodé de fils d'or, plus
gros à l'empièecement.
Grand col doublé en
taupe très souple.*

*Coat of taupe Chantilly
lace re-embroidered in
gold. Shirred yoke, large
collar lined with mole.*

GABRIELLE CHANEL

LES GRANDES
ÉLÉGANCES

*Manteau du soir, en satin noir
broché de roses « laque », à
feuillages d'or, doublé de mousseline de soie «laque» se voyant
de côté et à l'ouverture du
devant. Col doublé et froncé
sur double pèlerine.*

*Evening coat of black satin
brocaded with lacquer red
roses with gold leaves, lined
with lacquer red mousseline
de soie visible at the side slits
and front opening. Collar
lined and shirred over a double cape.*

CHÉRUIT

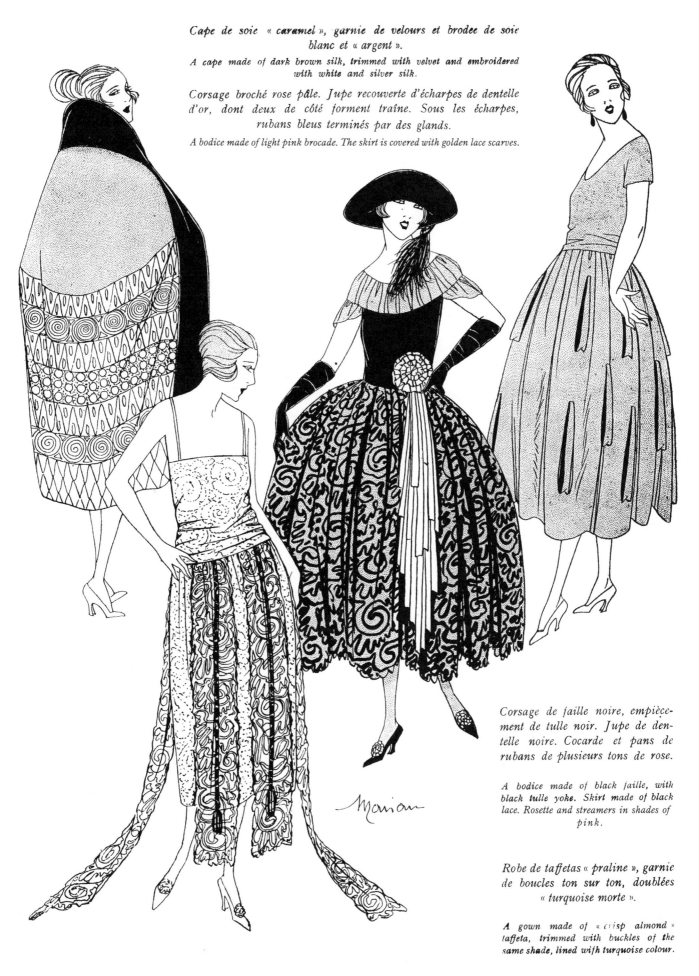

Cape de soie « caramel », garnie de velours et brodee de soie blanc et « argent ».

A cape made of dark brown silk, trimmed with velvet and embroidered with white and silver silk.

Corsage broché rose pâle. Jupe recouverte d'écharpes de dentelle d'or, dont deux de côté forment traîne. Sous les écharpes, rubans bleus terminés par des glands.

A bodice made of light pink brocade. The skirt is covered with golden lace scarves.

Corsage de faille noire, empièce-ment de tulle noir. Jupe de dentelle noire. Cocarde et pans de rubans de plusieurs tons de rose.

A bodice made of black faille, with black tulle yoke. Skirt made of black lace. Rosette and streamers in shades of pink.

Robe de taffetas « praline », garnie de boucles ton sur ton, doublées « turquoise morte ».

A gown made of « crisp almond » taffeta, trimmed with buckles of the same shade, lined with turquoise colour.

The outfits of Mademoiselle JEANNE PROVOST

in *Les Ailes Brisées* [The Broken Wings] at the Vaudeville

∎

Creations by

Jeanne LANVIN

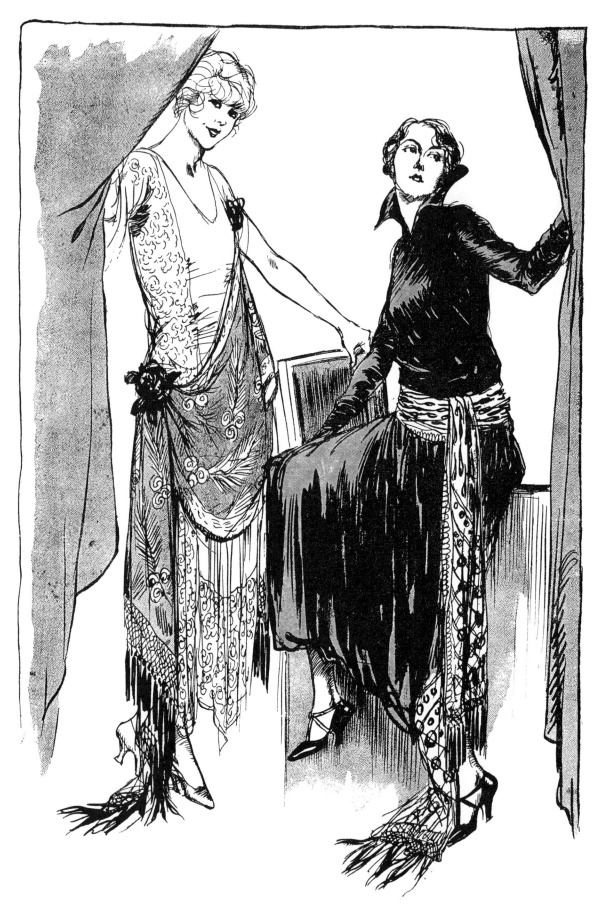

*Le nom seul de cette robe ne vous
fait-il pas rêver ? Elle est en Souffle
de soie et combien joliment drapée
d'une merveilleuse écharpe Batik.!*

A gown made of Souffle de soie
and lace with a batik scarf.

*N'est-elle pas somptueuse sur
cette robe de velours noir, cette
longue et souple écharpe bleu,
blanc, vert avec galon argenté ?*

*A gown made of black velvet;
blue, white and green scarf.*

BATIK SCARVES FROM THE HOUSE OF BIANCHINI, FÉRIER.

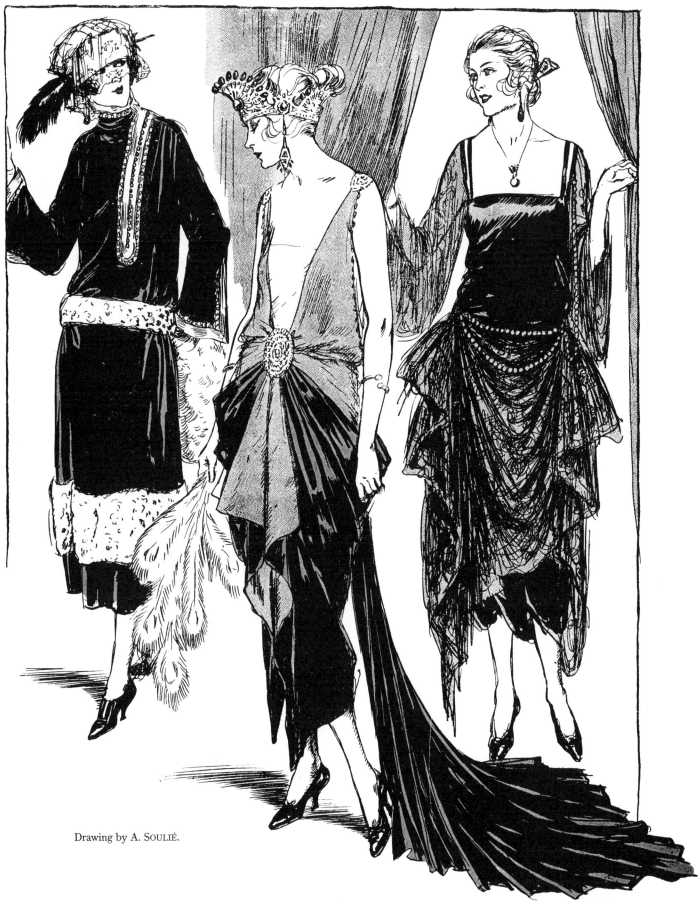

Drawing by A. SOULIÉ.

PERSANE

Robe d'après-midi, en drap noir.
Corsage et bas de manche garnis de
broderie et de piqûres grises. Ceinture
et bas de jupe de petit astrakan gris.

An afternoon gown made of black cloth.
Bodice and lower-part of the sleeves trimmed
with embroidery and grey stitches. Belt and
lower part of the skirt made of astrakhan.

SÉMIRAMIS

Robe du soir, en satin noir. Corsage de
satin bleu. Jupe de satin noir drapée et
retenue au corsage par un motif de diamants
blancs. Epaulette brodée de diamants blancs.

An evening gown made of black satin. Blue
satin bodice. Draped skirt made of black satin.
Shoulder straps embroidered with rhinestones.

PHRYNÉ

Robe de dîner, en dentelle
noire drapée sur fourreau
de crêpe satin noir.
Collier de perles «jade».

A dinner gown, made of
black lace draped over black
crepe satin. Necklace of
jade beads.

CREATIONS BY WORTH

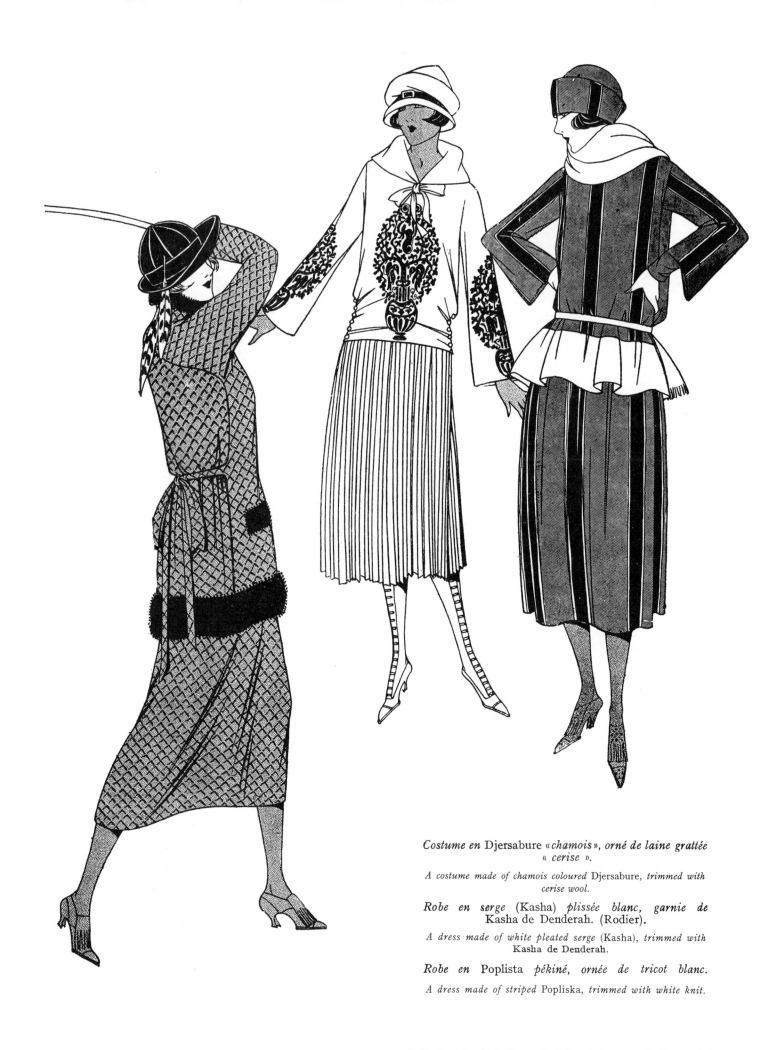

Costume en Djersabure *«chamois», orné de laine grattée « cerise ».*

A costume made of chamois coloured Djersabure, *trimmed with cerise wool.*

Robe en serge (Kasha) *plissée blanc, garnie de* Kasha de Denderah. (Rodier).

A dress made of white pleated serge (Kasha), *trimmed with* Kasha de Denderah.

Robe en Poplista *pékiné, ornée de tricot blanc.*

A dress made of striped Popliska, *trimmed with white knit.*

GOLFING AT ST. CLOUD

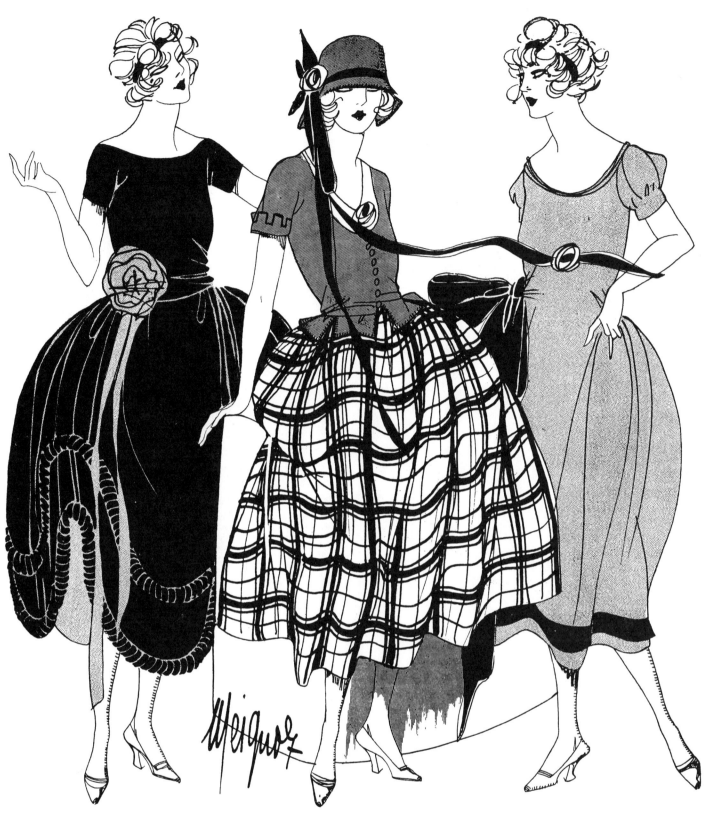

Creations from the House of

NICOLE GROULT

29, rue d'Anjou.

AMANDA
Robe en taffetas « bleu Nattier », doublée de satin « rose Chine » cocarde du même ton.

A dress made of Nattier blue taffeta, lined with Chinese pink satin; matching rosette.

DONJON
Jupe en tuffetas écossais noir et blanc. Casaque en taffetas « bleu roi », brodé de taffetas noir. Chapeau en taffetas « bleu roi », brodé noir. Petites roses.

A skirt made of black and white plaid taffeta. Overblouse made of royal blue taffeta, embroidered with black taffeta. Hat made of royal blue taffeta, embroidered in black. Small roses.

CHENONCEAU
Robe en taffetas rose «ibis». Bord du décolleté et biais du bas de la jupe en velours bleu Nattier. Large ruban du même ton au côté de la robe.

A dress made of « ibis » coloured pink taffeta. Bodice and skirt edged with Nattier blue velvet. Wide matching ribbon, on side.

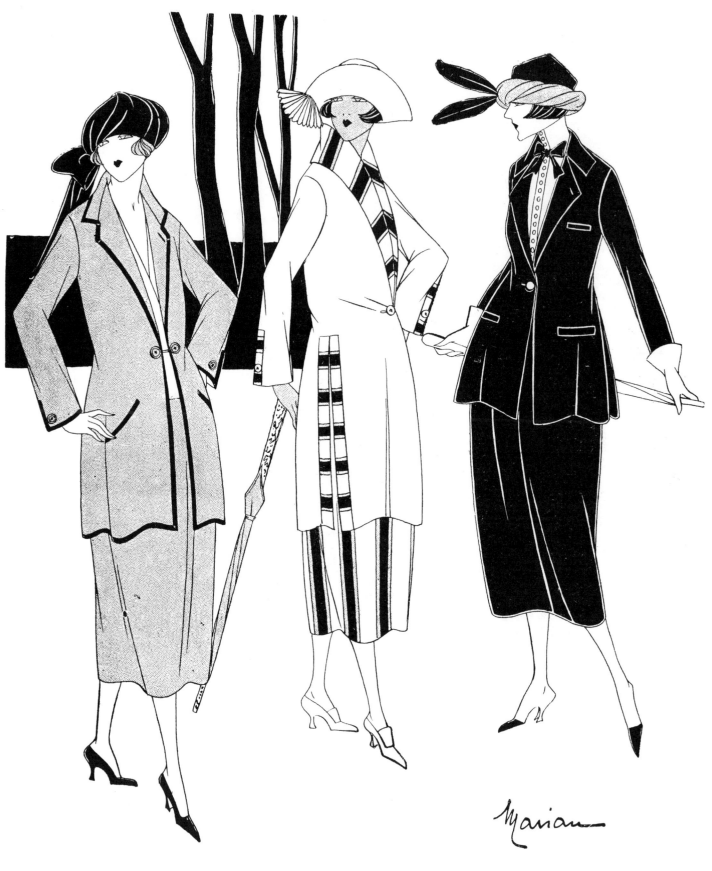

WE'RE WEARING SUITS MORE THAN EVER

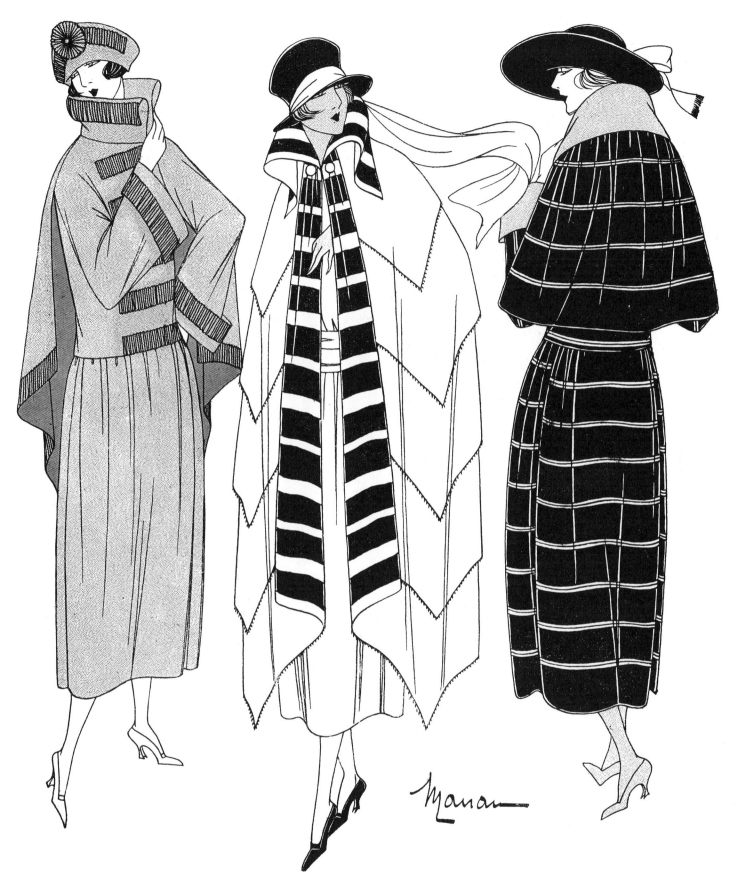

Manteau en Perllaine
« glycine », orné de
galon gaufré.

A coat of wisteria coloured
Perllaine, *trimmed with
pleated braid.*

Cape en serge « gris
argent », garnie de
velours pékiné.

*A silver grey serge cape,
trimmed with striped vel-
vet.*

Manteau de lainage
écossais, garni de cuir
rouge « laque ».

*A coat of plaid wool,
trimmed with lacquer red
leather.*

FOR GOING TO THE RACES AT DISTANT TRACKS

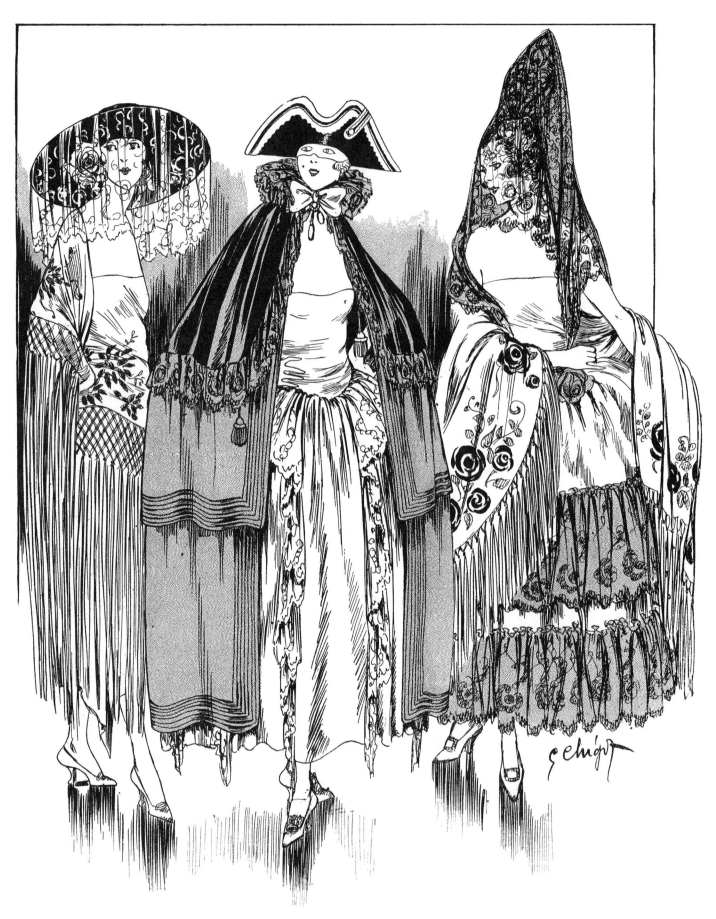

Robe faite d'un châle espagnol mauve, brodé pourpre.

A gown made of a mauve Spanish shawl, embroidered in purple.

Domino vénitien en tissu d'argent avec petite cape de soie violette, ouvert sur une robe « géranium ».

A Venetian domino made of silver tissue ; short cape made of violet silk, over a « geranium » coloured gown.

Robe en satin pourpre et dentelle espagnole, grand châle «argent», brodé rouge et violet.

A gown made of purple satin and Spanish lace, large silver shawl, red and violet embroidery.

AT THE OPERA BALL (June 25)

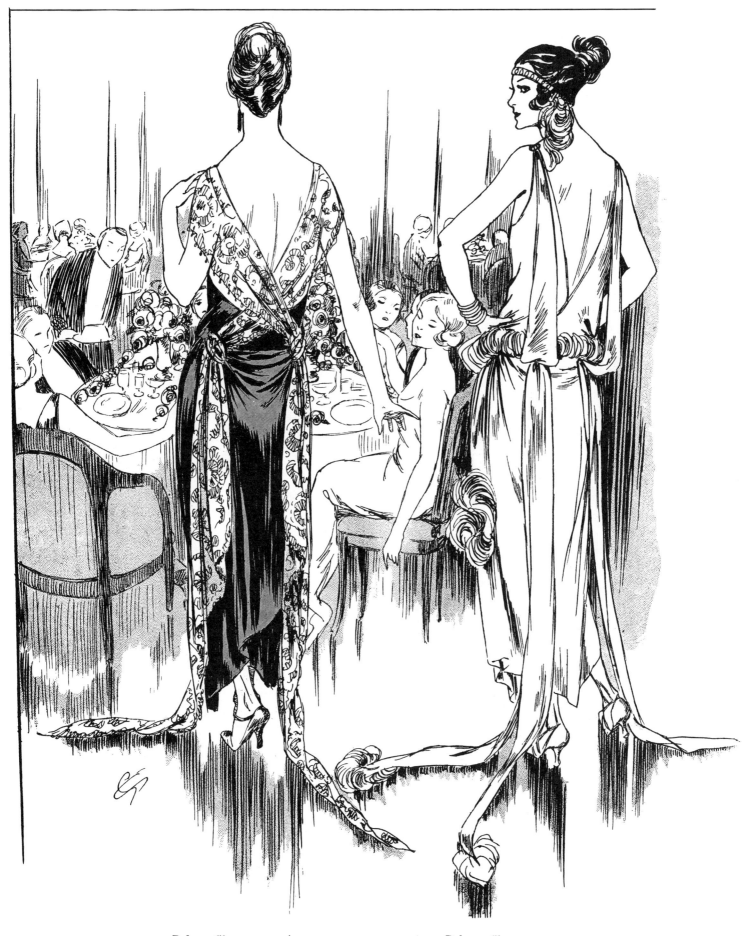

Robe en Charmeuse noire
et dentelle d'or.

Black **Charmeuse** (*satin*) *and*
golden lace

Robe en Charmeuse *mauve*
et plumes du ton.

Mauve Charmeuse (*satin*) *and*
matching feathers.

SATURDAY DINNERS AT THE CERCLE INTERALLIÉ

ARE FASHION CONTESTS

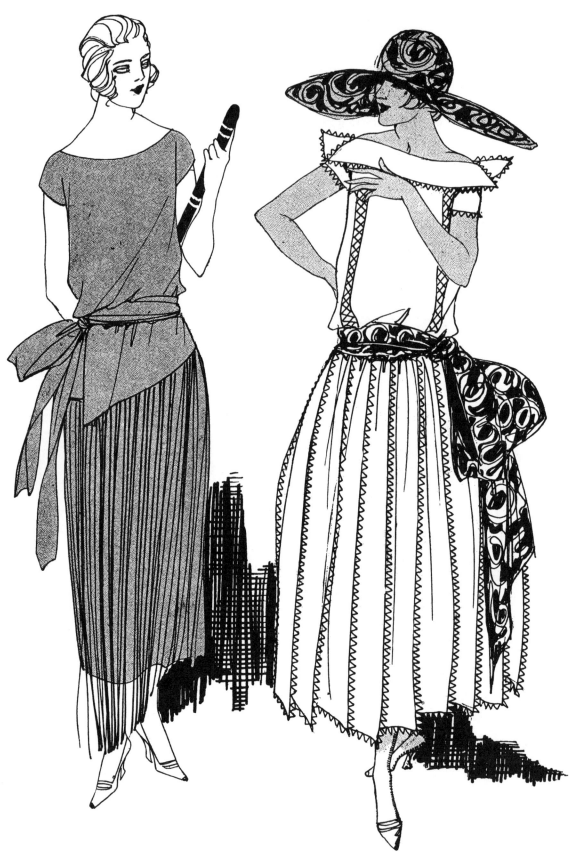

*Robe de satin gris;
tunique de frange de
soie même ton.*

*A dress made of grey
satin; tunic made of the
same shaded silk fringe.*

*Robe d'organdi blanc. Jupe faite de panneaux
dentelés. Petits revers formant l'encolure « bateau »;
large ceinture de mousseline imprimée.*

*A white organdy dress. Skirt made of jagged-edged panels.
Small collar forming bateau neck. Wide printed chiffon sash.*

The Outfits worn by Mlle. SYBIL FLORIAN

in Le Bonheur à 5 sous [Happiness for 5 Cents] at the Comédie-Montaigne.

CREATIONS BY TOLLMANN

35, Rue de Miromesnil, 35

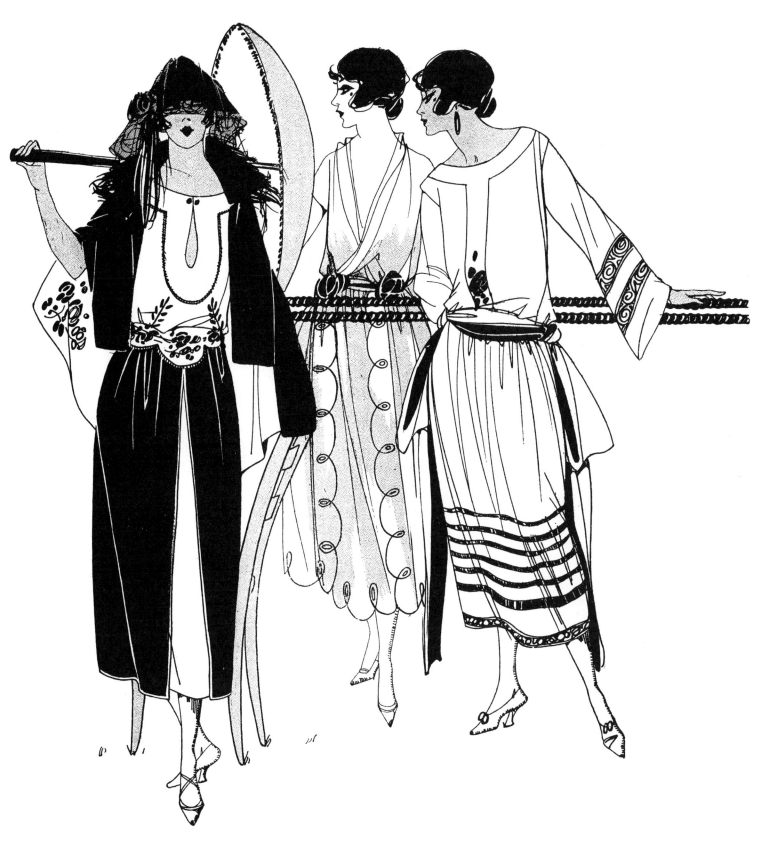

Robe trois pièces en drap noir et crêpe marocain blanc. Broderies chinoises et col de singe.

Black cloth and white crêpe marocain, **Chinese embroidery, monkey-fur collar.**

Robe en organdi rose sur fond « canard ».

Pink organdy over duck coloured slip.

Robe en crêpe marocain blanc et mousseline. Broderies persanes.

White crêpe marocain and chiffon. Persian embroidery.

THE OUTFITS OF MLLE. SUZY DANTÈS

in *Un Ange Passa* [An Angel Passed], at the Potinière.

CREATIONS BY JEAN PATOU, 7, Rue Saint-Florentin.

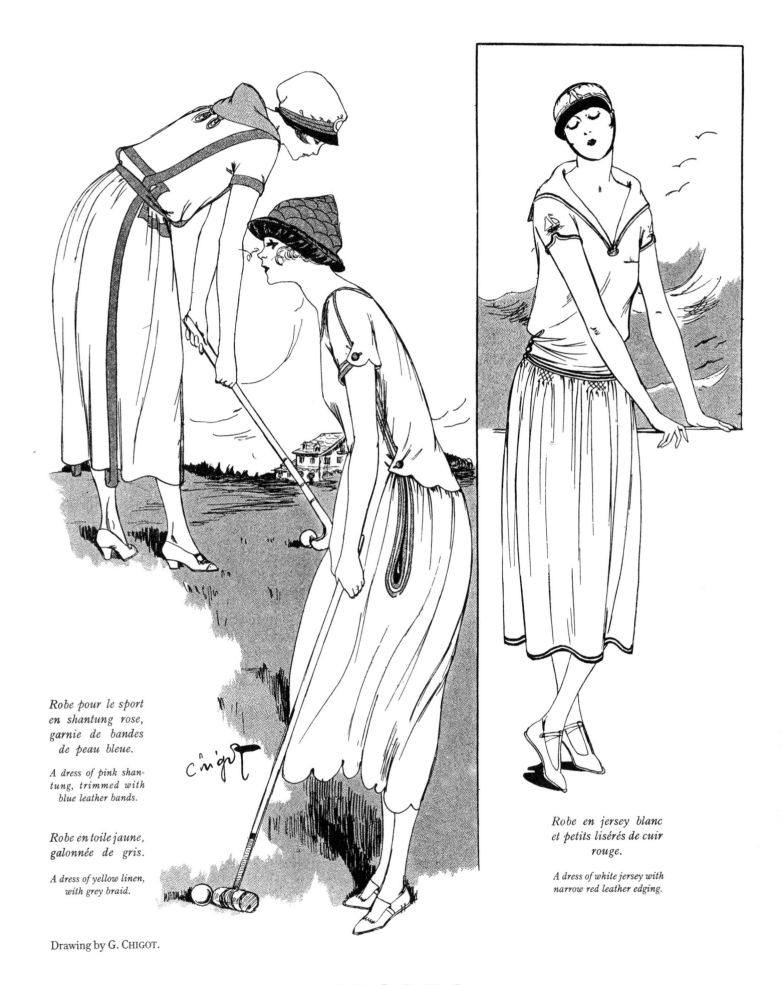

Robe pour le sport en shantung rose, garnie de bandes de peau bleue.

A dress of pink shantung, trimmed with blue leather bands.

Robe en toile jaune, galonnée de gris.

A dress of yellow linen, with grey braid.

Drawing by G. CHIGOT.

Robe en jersey blanc et petits lisérés de cuir rouge.

A dress of white jersey with narrow red leather edging.

SPORTS

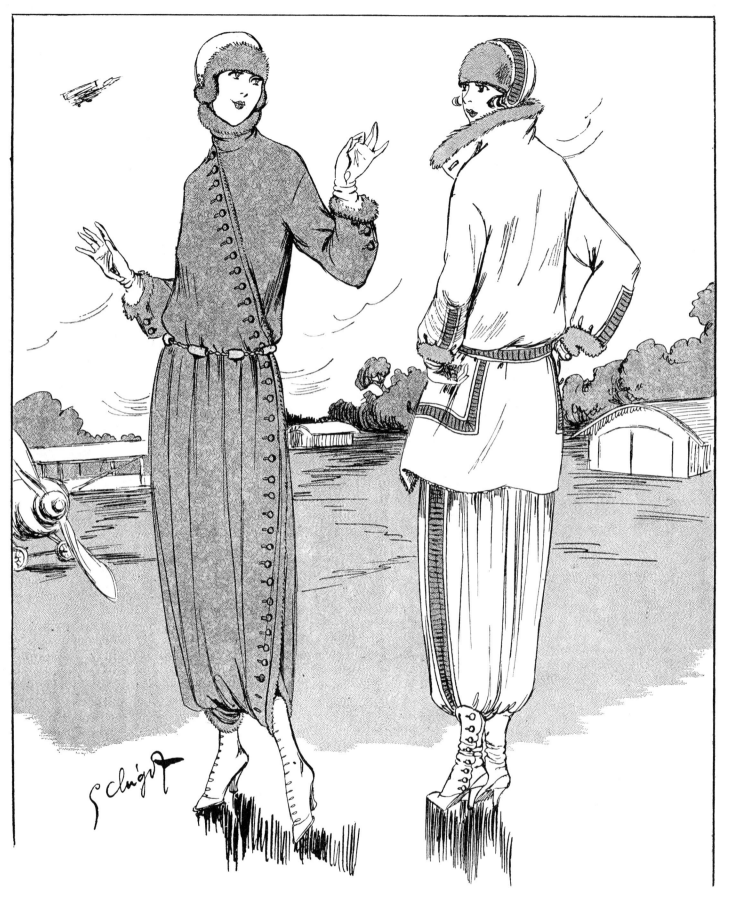

*Combinaison pour mettre sur une robe,
en peau souple havane, boutonnée
de cuir et garnie de castor.*

A flying suit to be worn over a dress and made of soft tobacco coloured
leather, with leather buttons and trimmed with beaver fur.

*Combinaison en Perllaine grise,
incrustée rouge. Cette combinaison peut
également se passer sur une robe.*

A flying suit made of grey Perllaine, with insets of
red leather.

Look how flying is attracting women! In fact, fashionable women no longer hesitate to receive
"baptism by air." It has become the fashion, the rage! Consequently, a special costume—practical,
warm and elegant—has become imperative. What do you think of these two? Without a doubt they
will conquer all the fashionable skies . . . Deauville, Trouville, etc.

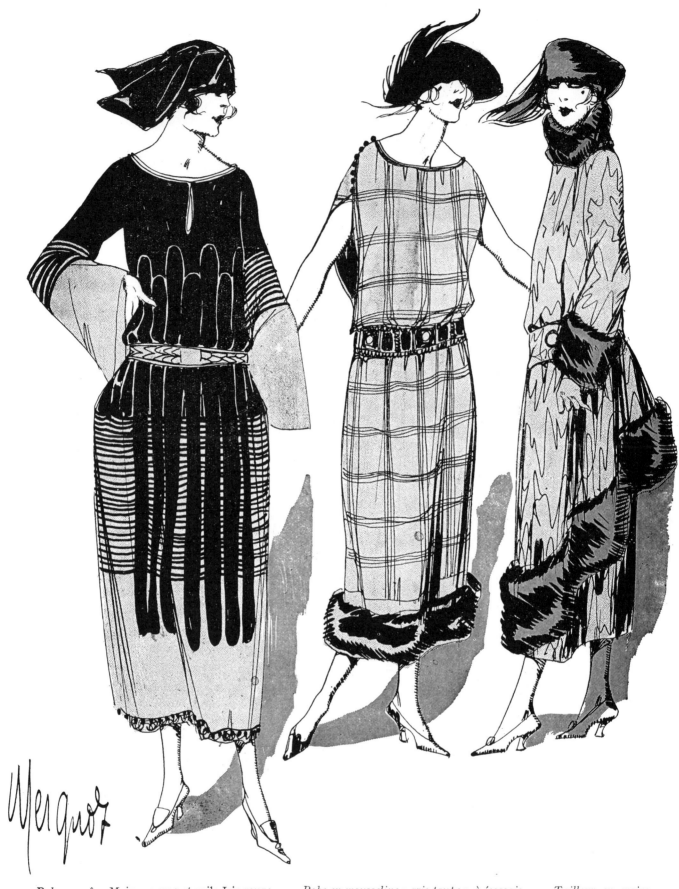

Robe en crêpe Majunga *noir et* voile Isis *rouge
garnie de galons de soie noire. Dessous dépassant
légèrement en dentelle noire. Ceinture de cuir.*

Black Majunga crape *and red*
Isis veil; *black silk braid. Leather belt.*

*Robe en mousseline « gris taupe » à écossais
de velours vert. Ceinture en broderie d'argent ēt
plaques de velours, ourlée de renard gris.*

*Grey chiffon, plaided in green velvet; silver
embroidered belt, grey fox hem.*

*Tailleur en moire
grise, ourlé de
renard gris.*

*Grey moiré suit,
grey fox edging.*

CREATIONS BY MARGAINE-LACROIX

19, Boulevard Haussmann

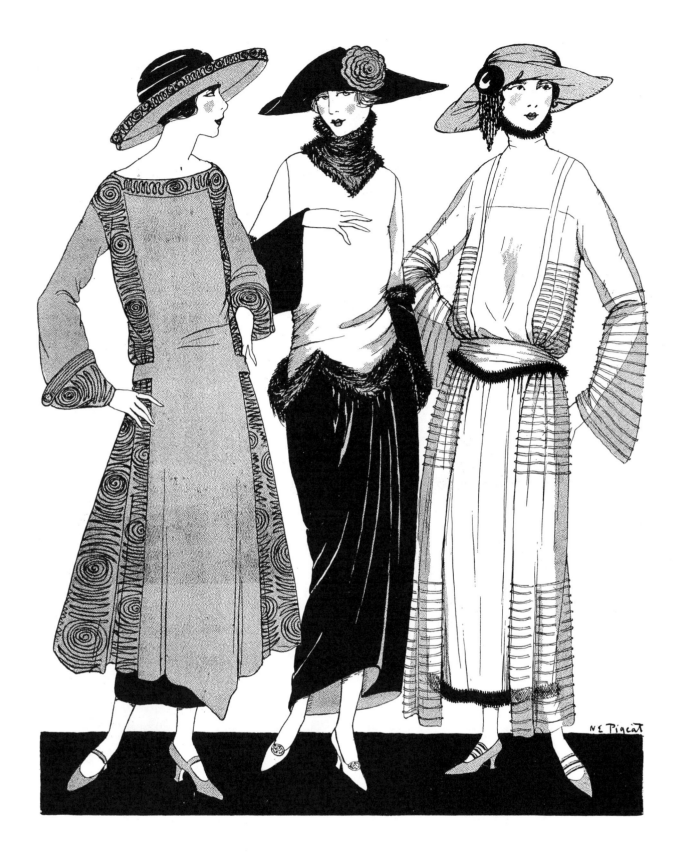

Aussi bien pour le matin que pour l'après-midi, on peut porter la robe de serge. Celle-ci est en forme. Le tablier se termine en pointe et les côtés de la robe, ainsi que les poignets, sont brodés de grosse soie « citron ».

A gown made of serge ; sides and cuffs embroidered with lemon coloured heavy silk.

En septembre, on peut encore sortir sans manteau, pourvu que la robe soit assez chaude, avec un peu de fourrure. Exemple : ce fourreau de velours vert assez foncé, sur lequel vient se draper un velours noir retenu aux hanches par un bourrelet de fourrure. Cette robe est assez élégante pour le thé.

A frock made of dark green velvet, with a drapery made of black velvet, held on the hips by a band of fur.

Pour le thé également et même pour un petit dîner de septembre, le troisième modèle ira à merveille. Il est en voile noir à panneaux garnis de très petits plis. Un peu de fourrure, naturellement, souligne le col et termine la jupe.

A dress made of black voile, with panels trimmed with tiny pleats. Fur on collar and on the hem of skirt.

SERGE, VELVET OR VOILE?

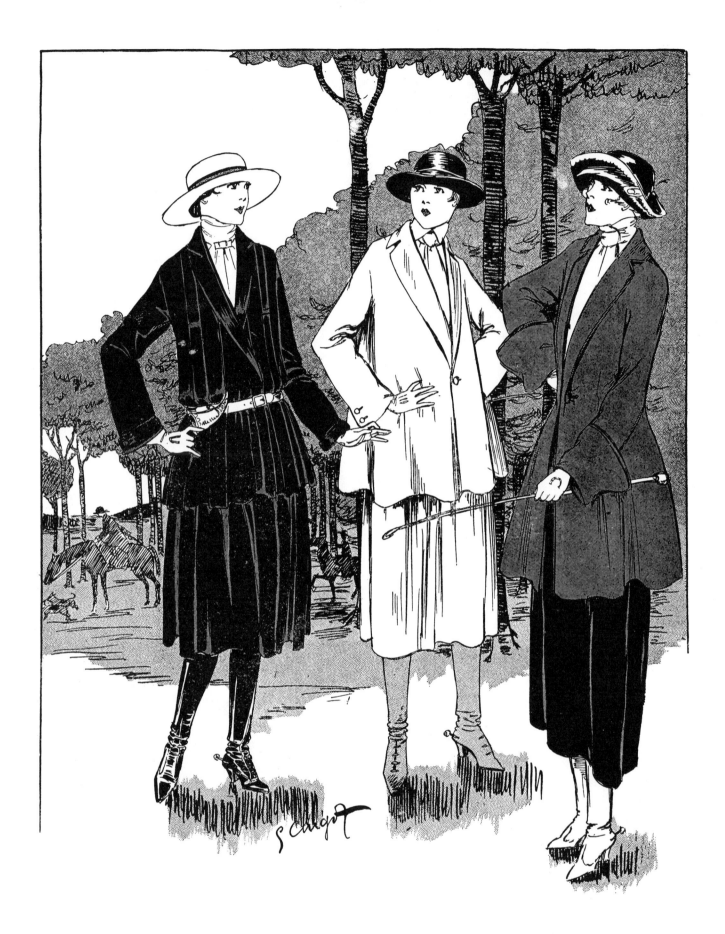

*Tailleur de chasse en velours
noir, ceinturé de daim blanc.*

■

*A hunting suit of black velvet,
with a white doeskin belt.*

*Tailleur en
peau grise.*

■

*A suit of
grey leather.*

Tailleur en Drapella
rouge et noir.

■

*A suit of red and
black* Drapella.

THE REOPENING OF THE HUNTING SEASON

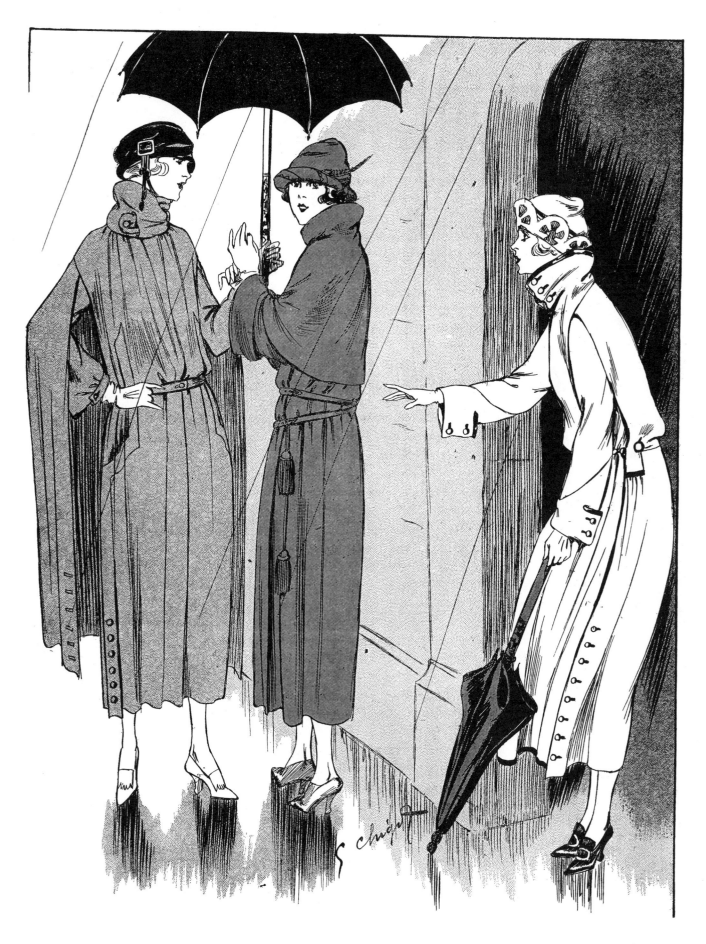

Manteau de pluie en Perlaine *grise.*

A coat for rainy days made of grey wool
(Perllaine).

Manteau en cuir souple « fumée ».

A coat of smoke coloured
soft leather.

*Manteau en lainage beige imperméabilisé,
garni de ciré marine.*

A coat of beige wool, trimmed with navy ciré.

IT'S RAINING, IT'S RAINING, MADAME! ...

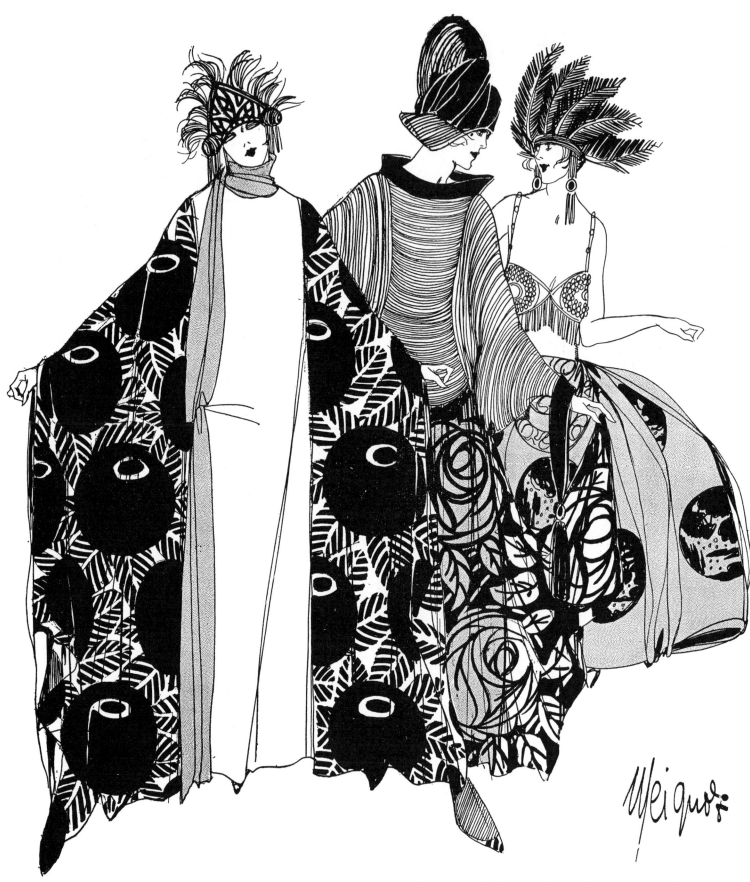

Manteau en Velours Van Dyck *rouge et lamé d'or à dessins de boules et feuillage en velours noir.*

Red Van Dyck *velvet.*
Golden lamé with black velvet balls and leaves.

Manteau en broderie d'or et lamé or, broché de roses et feuillage en velours « corail ».

Golden embroidery and golden lamé, with roses and leaves made of coral velvet.

Robe en crêpe Athénien *bleu ancien à dessins formant paysages (La Nuit étoilée) garni de rubans et dentelle d'argent.*

Antique blue Athenian *crêpe, with black pleated and embroidered starry-night designs, ribbons and silver lace trim.*

THE PARADE OF SILKS IN THE REVUE AT THE CASINO DE PARIS IS OF A RARE SUMP-
TUOUSNESS. THESE COSTUMES, EXECUTED AFTER SKETCHES BY ZINOVIEV, ARE MADE UP IN
THE BEAUTIFUL FABRICS OF F. DUCHARNE, OF LYONS.

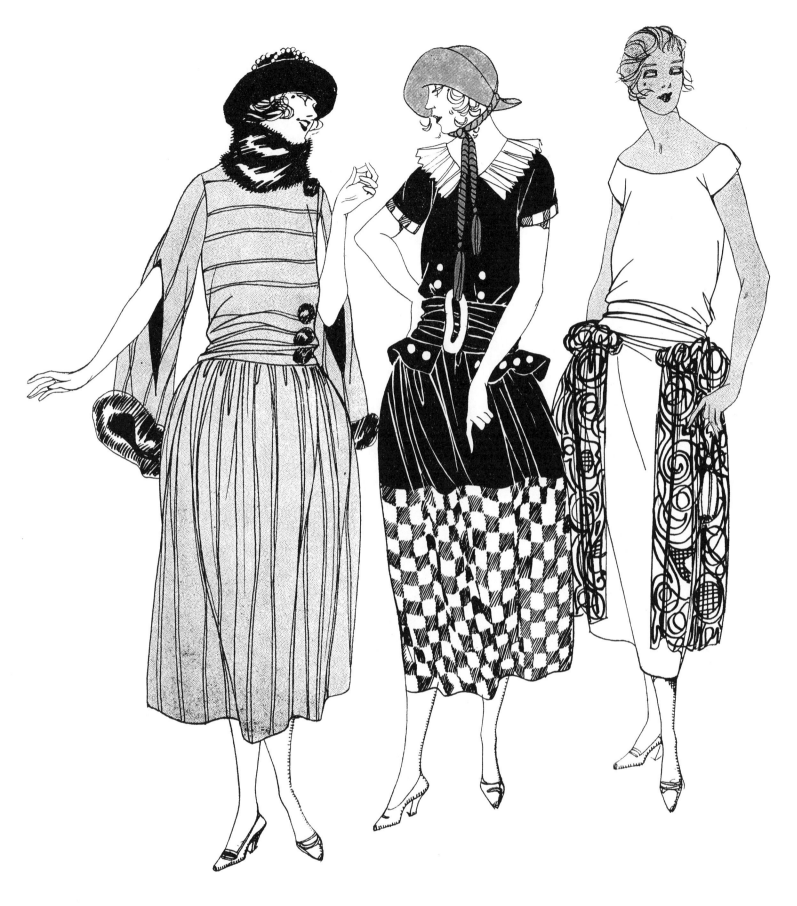

Robe en serge (Kasha) *beige, de deux tons pékinés, doublée de* crêpe Marie-Louise *« rouge piqueur » et ourlée de skungs.*

A gown made in two shades of beige serge (Kasha), lined with red crêpe Marie-Louise and edged with skunk fur.

Robe en serge (Kasha) *noire et lainage* (Dialisse) *à carreaux noirs et blancs ; boucle d'acier poli.*

A gown made of black serge (Kasha) and wool (Dialisse), **with** black **and** white squares; steel buckle.

Robe en satin Windsor *« neige » et jersey. Dentelle rouge « drapeau ».*

A gown made of snow coloured satin Windsor and jersey. Flag red lace.

The Outfits Worn in *Si que je s'rais roi?* [So I'm King?] at the Capucines.

CREATIONS BY POIRET

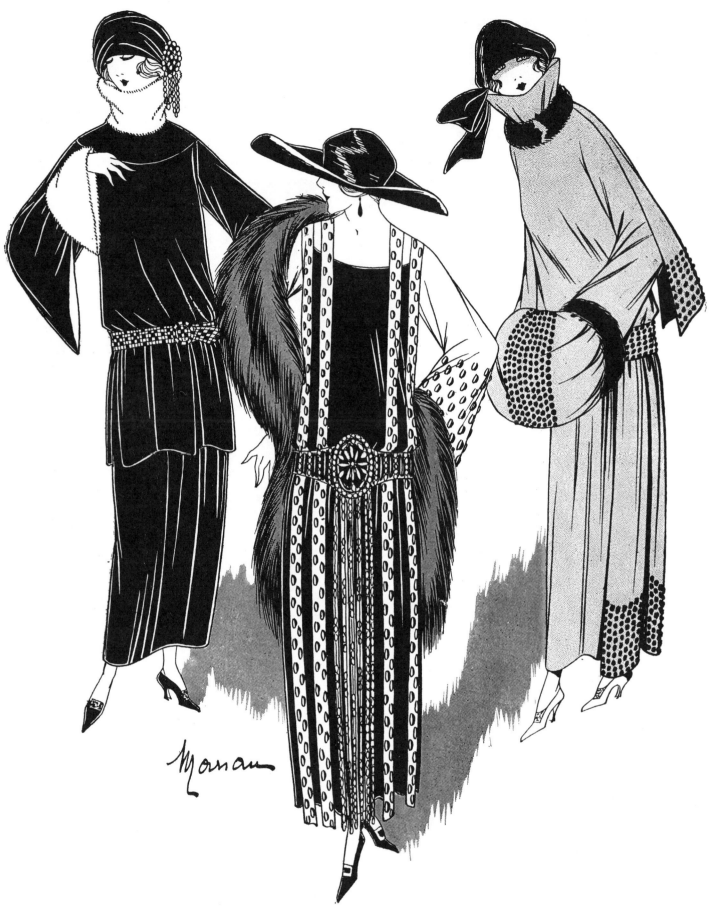

Costume de velours Van Dyck
noir, orné d'hermine ; ceinture
de jais noir et blanc.

Robe de crêpe Athénien noir
et « bois de rose », garnie de
perles « bois » et noires.

Manteau de Perllaine « gris nuage »,
orné de loutre et perlé de jais ; manchon
assorti au manteau.

Black Van Dyck velvet,
ermine fur. Black and white
jet belt.

Black and « bois de rose » coloured
Athenian crepe ; wooden coloured
and black beads.

Cloud coloured grey Perllaine coat,
otter fur and jet beads. Muff to match.

THREE DRESSES I WOULD LIKE FOR PAYING VISITS

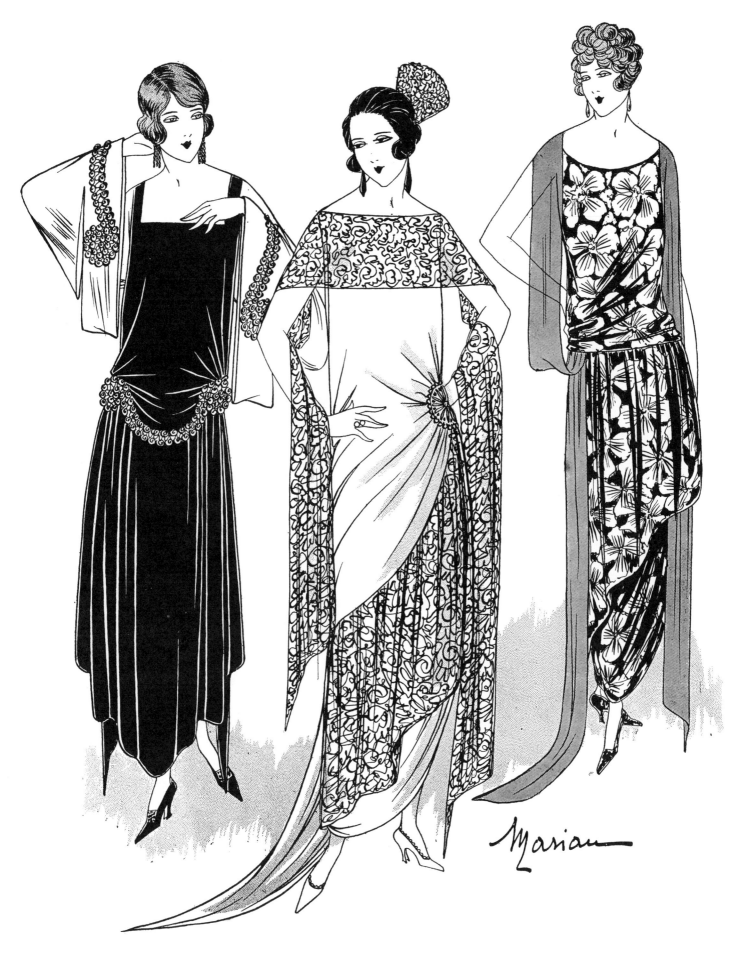

Robe de crêpe Romain *noir ; manches de voile blanc, ornées de coquillages nacrés.*

Robe du soir en velours Somptueux *« neige » ornée de dentelle d'argent.*

Robe de brocart noir et « acier » ; panneaux de mousseline « rouge laque ».

Crêpe Roman; *white voile sleeves with mother-of-pearl shells.*

White Somptueux velvet ; *silver lace.*

Black and steel coloured brocade; lacquer red chiffon panels.

THREE GOWNS THAT WOULD PLEASE ME FOR GOING OUT IN THE EVENING

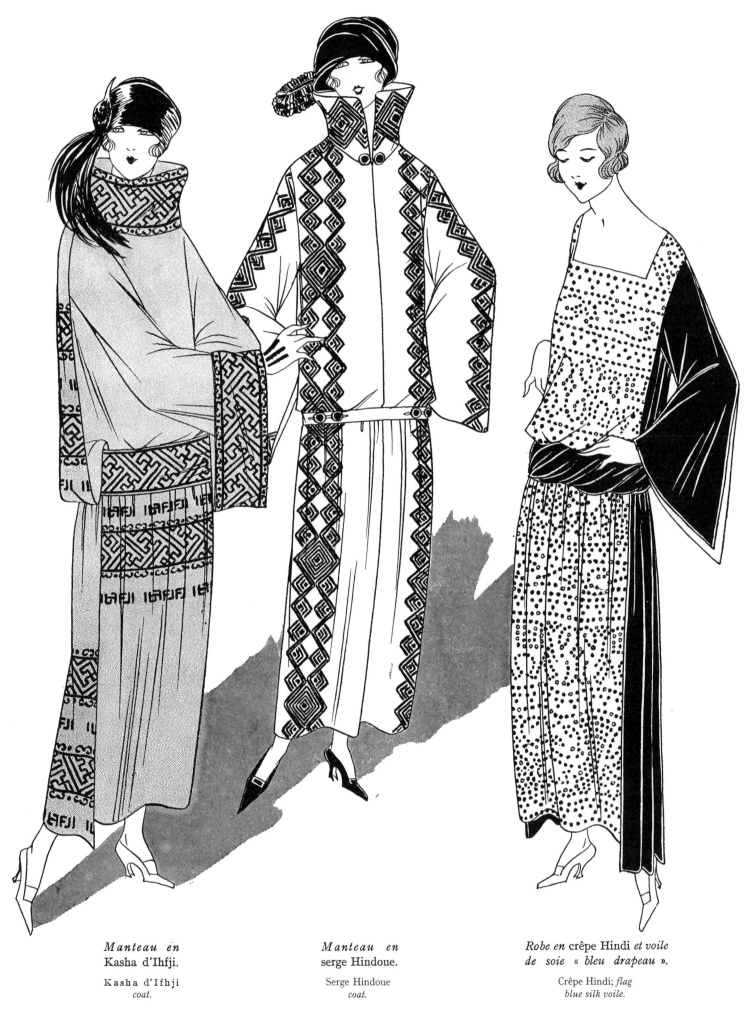

Manteau en
Kasha d'Ihfji.

Kasha d'Ifhji
coat.

Manteau en
serge Hindoue.

Serge Hindoue
coat.

Robe en crêpe Hindi *et voile
de soie « bleu drapeau ».*

Crêpe Hindi; *flag
blue silk voile.*

NEW FABRICS WILL BLOOM IN THE NEW SEASON

These are from RODIER

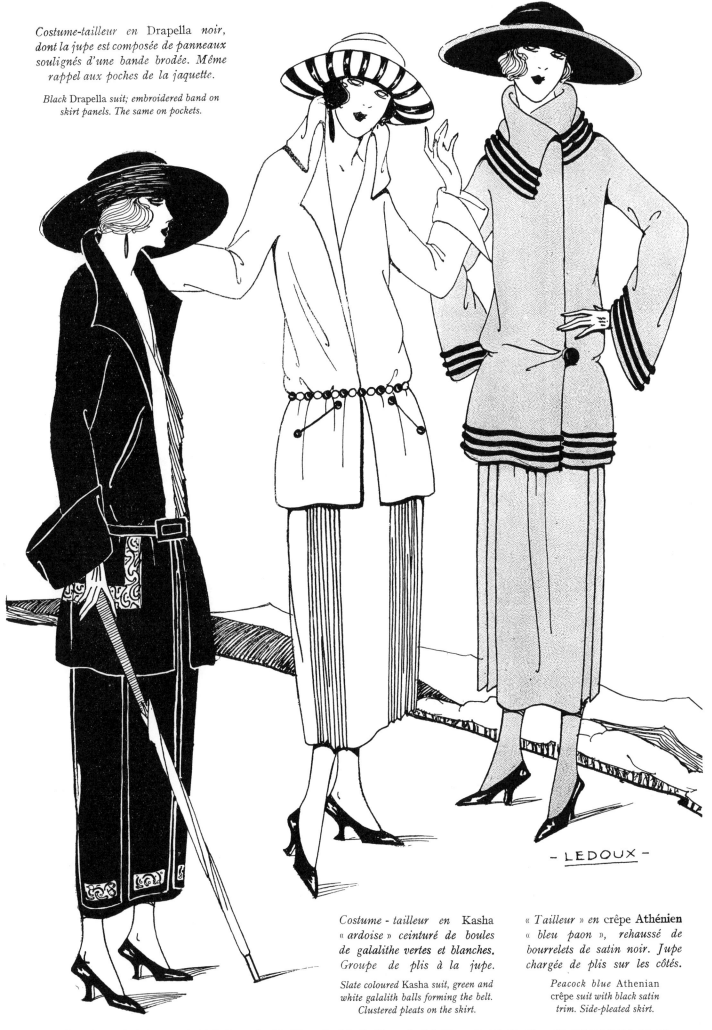

Costume-tailleur en Drapella noir, dont la jupe est composée de panneaux soulignés d'une bande brodée. Même rappel aux poches de la jaquette.

Black Drapella suit; embroidered band on skirt panels. The same on pockets.

Costume - tailleur en Kasha « ardoise » ceinturé de boules de galalithe vertes et blanches. Groupe de plis à la jupe.

Slate coloured Kasha suit, green and white galalith balls forming the belt. Clustered pleats on the skirt.

« Tailleur » en crêpe Athénien « bleu paon », rehaussé de bourrelets de satin noir. Jupe chargée de plis sur les côtés.

Peacock blue Athenian crêpe suit with black satin trim. Side-pleated skirt.

— LEDOUX —

WAISTLINES ARE LESS AND LESS DEFINED

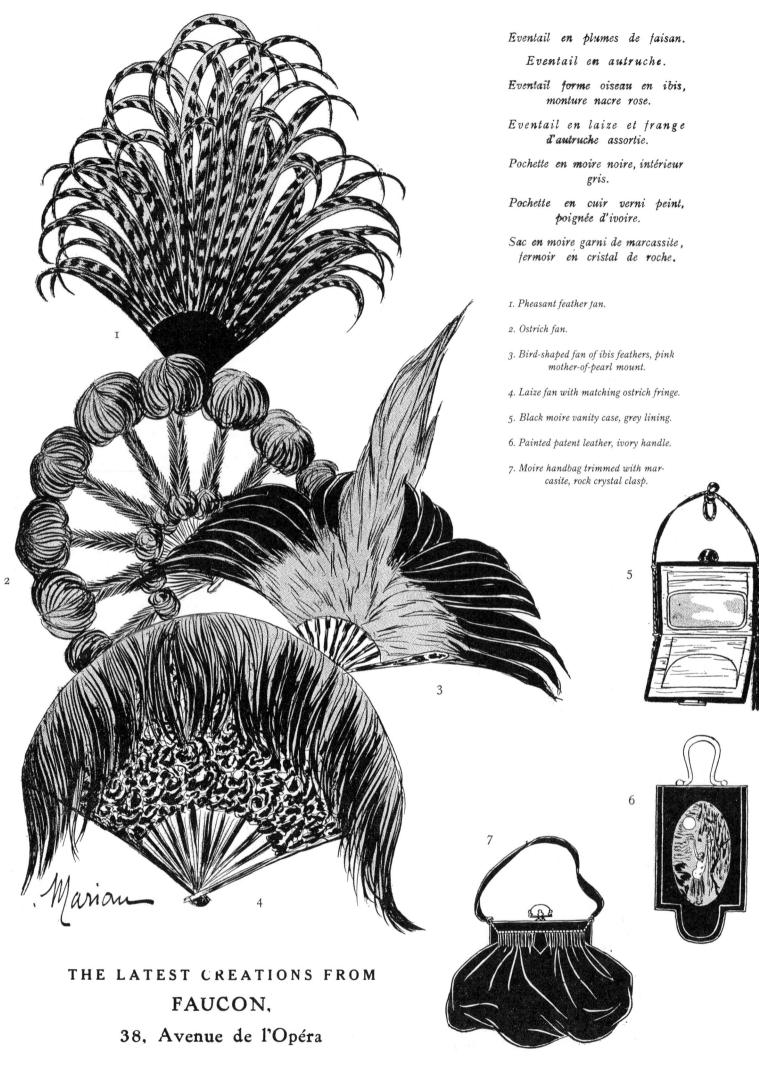

Eventail en plumes de faisan.

Eventail en autruche.

Eventail forme oiseau en ibis,
monture nacre rose.

Eventail en laize et frange
d'autruche assortie.

Pochette en moire noire, intérieur
gris.

Pochette en cuir verni peint,
poignée d'ivoire.

Sac en moire garni de marcassite,
fermoir en cristal de roche.

1. Pheasant feather fan.

2. Ostrich fan.

3. Bird-shaped fan of ibis feathers, pink
mother-of-pearl mount.

4. Laize fan with matching ostrich fringe.

5. Black moire vanity case, grey lining.

6. Painted patent leather, ivory handle.

7. Moire handbag trimmed with mar-
casite, rock crystal clasp.

**THE LATEST CREATIONS FROM
FAUCON,
38, Avenue de l'Opéra**

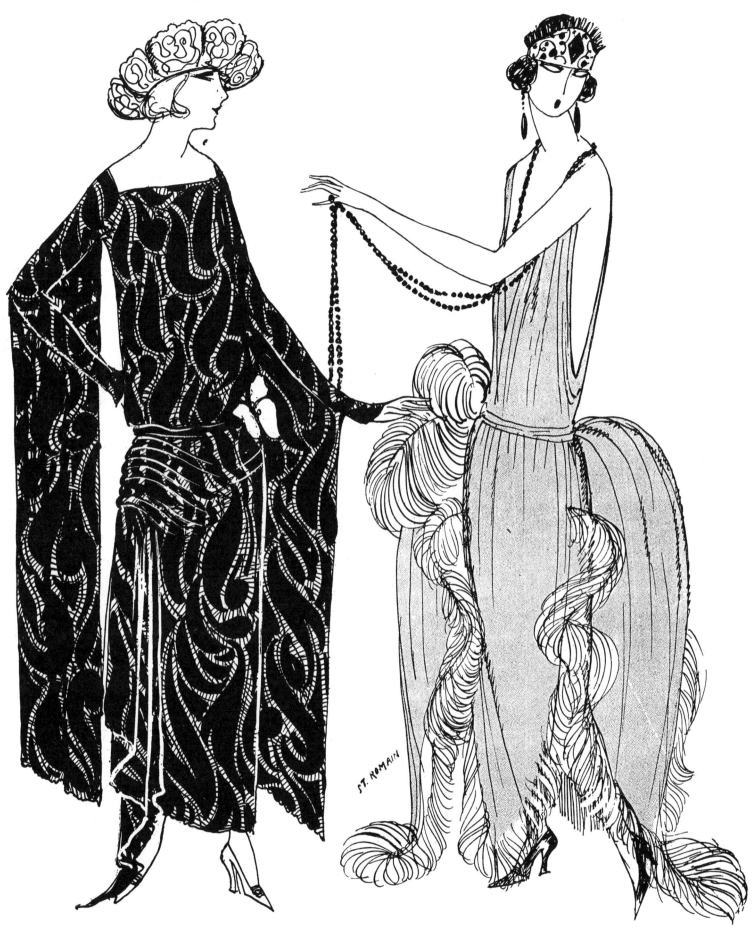

Fourreau de lamé « acier. » Robe drapée et longues manches de dentelle teinte « tango ». Ceinture « acier » et roses blanches de côté:

Steel lame frock ; draped gown and tango coloured lace long sleeves. Steel belt and white roses by side.

Fond de Salammbô « acier » et rose. Dessus de tulle vert de deux tons; plumes vertes dessinant les pointes. Pouf de plumes de côté.

Steel coloured and pink Salammbô slip. Tulle overdress of two shades of green; green feathers.

IN THE REVIVAL OF *LE MARQUIS DE PRIOLA* **AT THE FRANÇAIS, MLLE.**
CÉCILE SOREL WEARS THESE TWO SUMPTUOUS OUTFITS SIGNED BY

MOLYNEUX

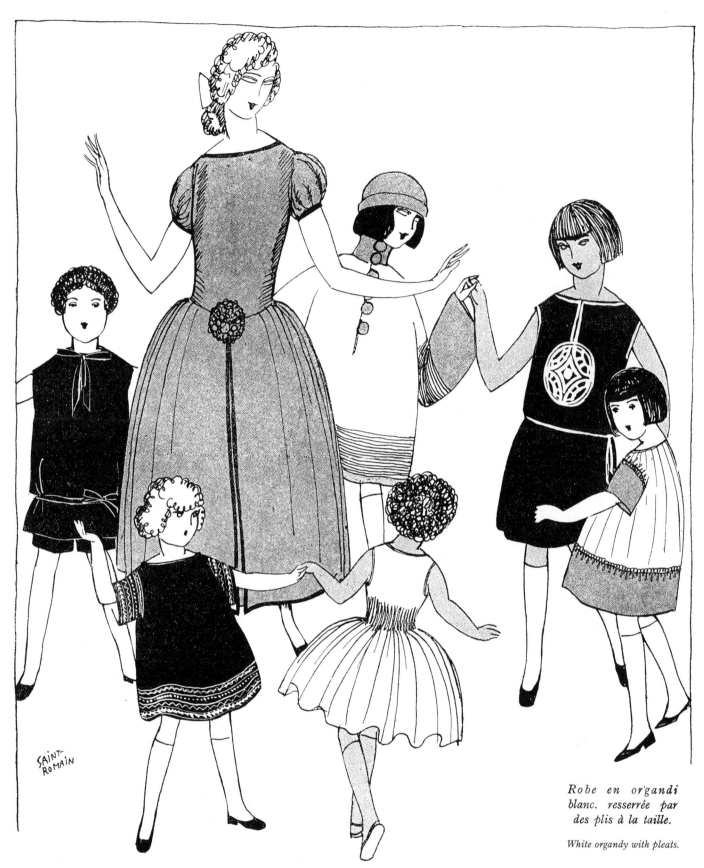

Robe en organdi blanc. resserrée par des plis à la taille.

White organdy with pleats.

Costume de tussor, pour garçonnet.	*Robe pour jeune fille, en taffetas, garnie de biais de même taffetas, plus foncé.*	*Petit paletot, en velours de laine bleu; col, poignets et boutons « cerise ».*	*Robe de* crêpe Marocain, *avec broderie de métal, ceinture nouée sur le côté.*	*Robe de* crêpe Marocain, *garnie de fine soutache.*	*Robe de* Crêpe satin noir, *garnie, dans le bas et aux manches, de broderie multicolore.*
Tussor costume for little boy.	*Taffeta gown, trimmed with same taffeta « biais », in a deeper shade.*	*Blue woolen velvet, cerise collar, wrist-bands and buttons.*	*Crêpe Marocain, metal embroidery; belt knotted at side.*	*Crêpe Marocain; fine soutache trim.*	*Black satin crêpe; multicolored embroidery on hem and sleeves.*

SOME PRETTY CREATIONS FROM ELINA
16, Rue Roquépine, 16

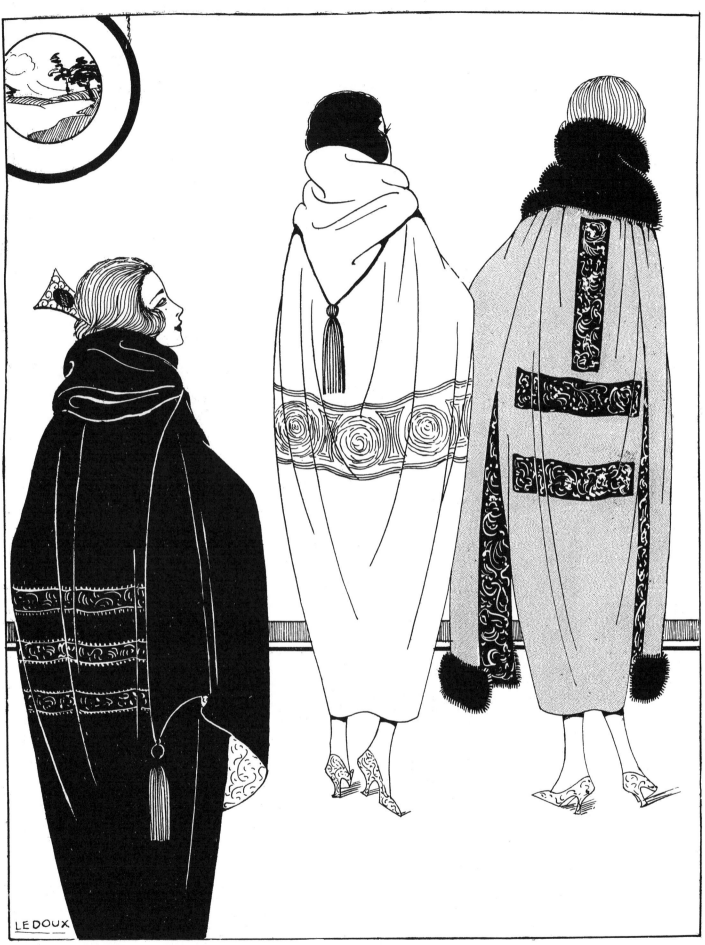

*Cape du soir, en satin Peplum noir,
doublée de satin « évêque ». Glands et
broderies de perles du même ton.*

Black satin Peplum, *lined with violet satin.
Matching tassels and bead embroidery.*

*Cape en moire indienne «dragée»,
brodée de fils d'argent. Gland
d'argent terminant le col pointu.*

Pink « moire indienne », *embroidered
with silver thread. Silver tassel.*

*Manteau du soir, en satin
Nessus « géranium »,
orné de kolinsky.*

Geranium coloured Nessus
satin ; kolinsky *fur.*

SOME CAPES

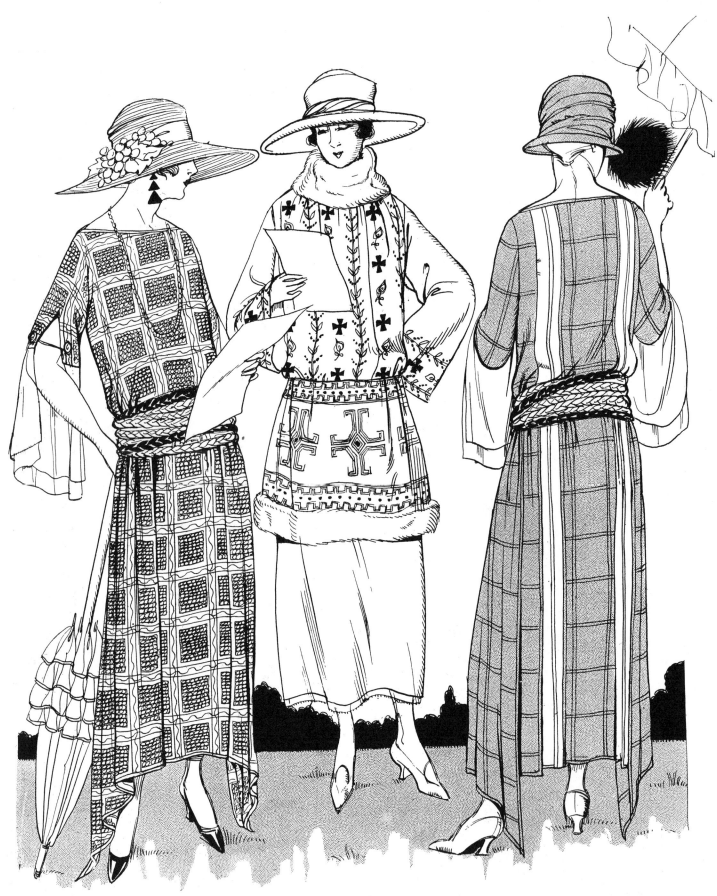

De PREMET, cette jolie robe de foulard blanc, «groseille» et noir; elle est garnie de mousseline de soie «groseille»; la ceinture faite de tresses en tissu des trois tons.

From Premet, a white, red currant and black foulard; red currant chiffon; braided cloth belt of the three shades.

Il a énormément de succès, ce modèle de crêpe Marocain blanc, joliment brodé et garni d'une façon si imprévue de «Pingouin»; il est signé: CHANEL.

White embroidered crêpe Marocain, trimmed with «Pingouin» signed "Chanel."

Dos de la robe nº 1 en foulard et mousseline de soie.

Back of the gown nº 1: foulard and chiffon.

PREMET AND CHANEL at the Chantilly Derby

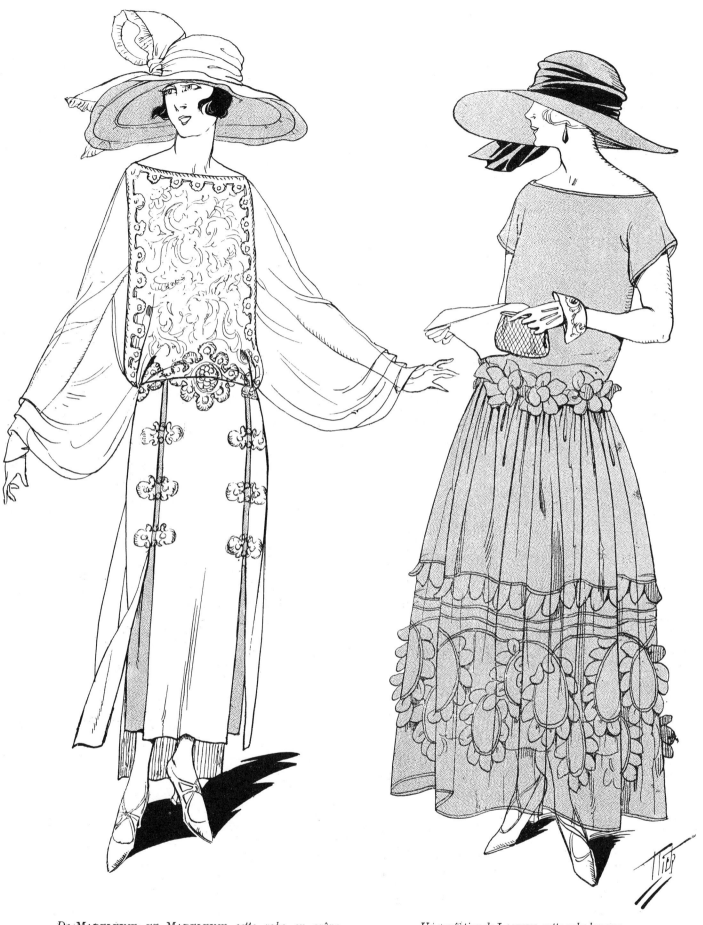

De MADELEINE ET MADELEINE *cette robe en* crêpe
Athénien *blanc, très joliment brodé de soie et fil de métal ;
la jupe est faite de panneaux s'ouvrant sur un fourreau
assorti ; larges manches en* crêpe Georgette.

From Madeleine and Madeleine, white Athenian crêpe with silk and
metal thread embroidery; skirt made of panels opening over a matching frock; wide sleeves of crêpe Georgette.

Une création de LANVIN, *cette robe longue
et vaporeuse, garnie de petits biais et
pétales découpés d'une grande légèreté ;
elle a été très remarquée au pesage.*

Narrow bias piping and cut-
out petals, from Lanvin.

MADELEINE AND MADELEINE, JEANNE LANVIN, at the Chantilly Derby

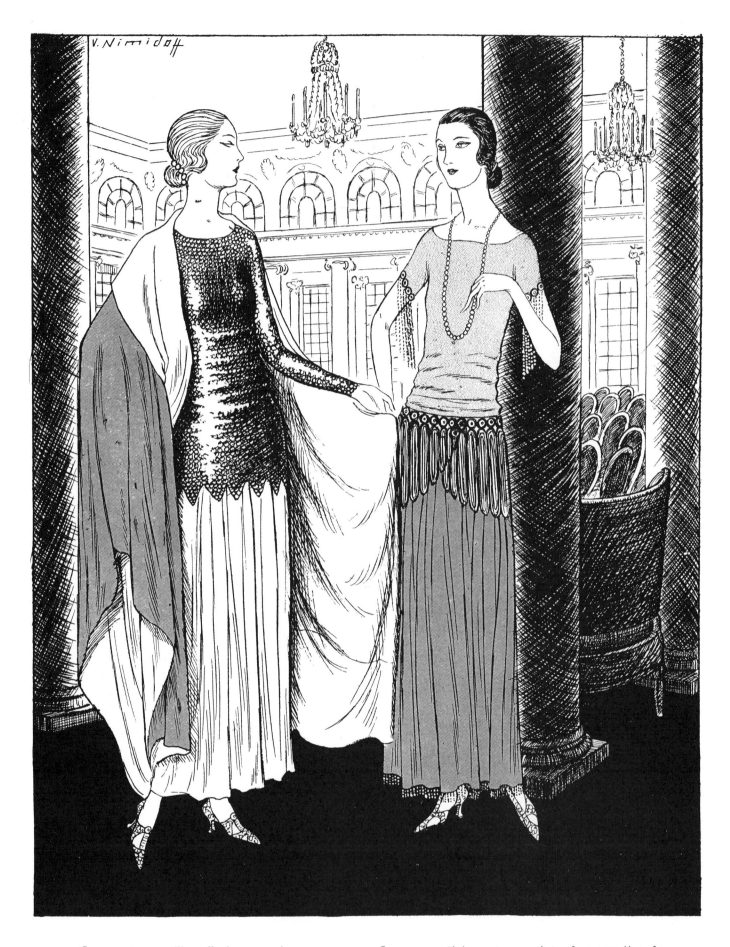

Casaque en mailles d'acier sur jupe de crêpe Romain blanc.

Steel netting overblouse; white crêpe Romain skirt.

Corsage en Fulgurante sur jupe de mousseline de soie. Ceinture et manches en franges de perles.

Fulgurante bodice; chiffon skirt. Beaded fringe sash and sleeves.

TWO POIRET GOWNS SEEN AT DEAUVILLE

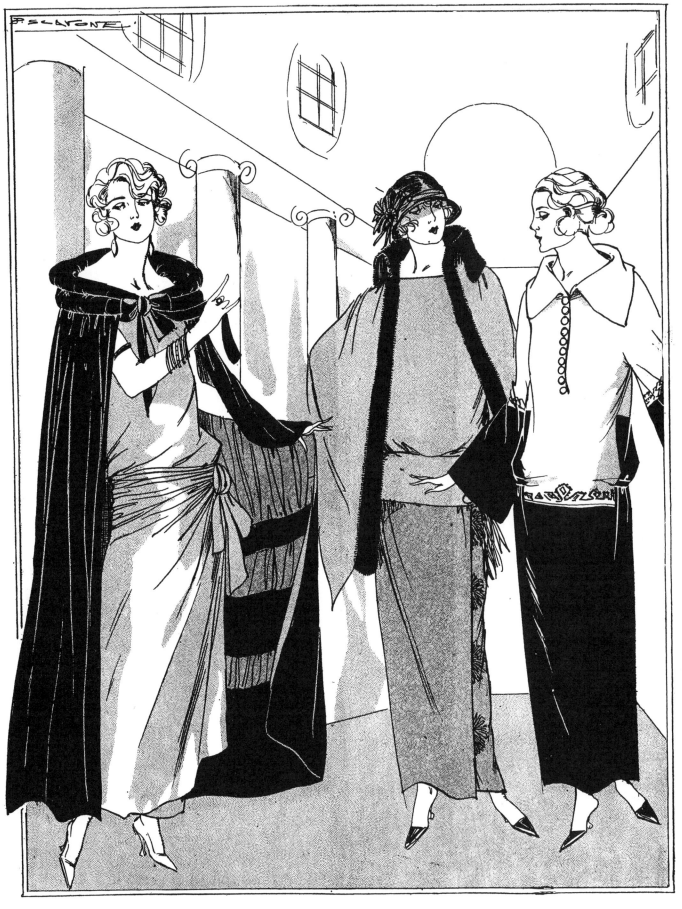

Cape en velours Sapho noir, doublé orange et robe de même velours que la doublure de la cape.

Black Sapho velvet, *orange lined.* **Gown** made of *same velvet as lining of cape.*

Trois-pièces un tissu façonné beige, garni de cocardes de daim et castor.

Beige fabric; rosettes of doeskin and beaver fur.

Robe en panne blanche et satin noir.

White velvet and black satin.

EVERY FRIDAY AT THE GRAND VATEL, THE MOST ELEGANT SPOT IN PARIS FOR TAKING TEA, CHARMING MANNEQUINS SHOW THE CREATIONS OF THE STARS OF COUTURE.

HERE ARE THOSE FROM LUCIEN LELONG

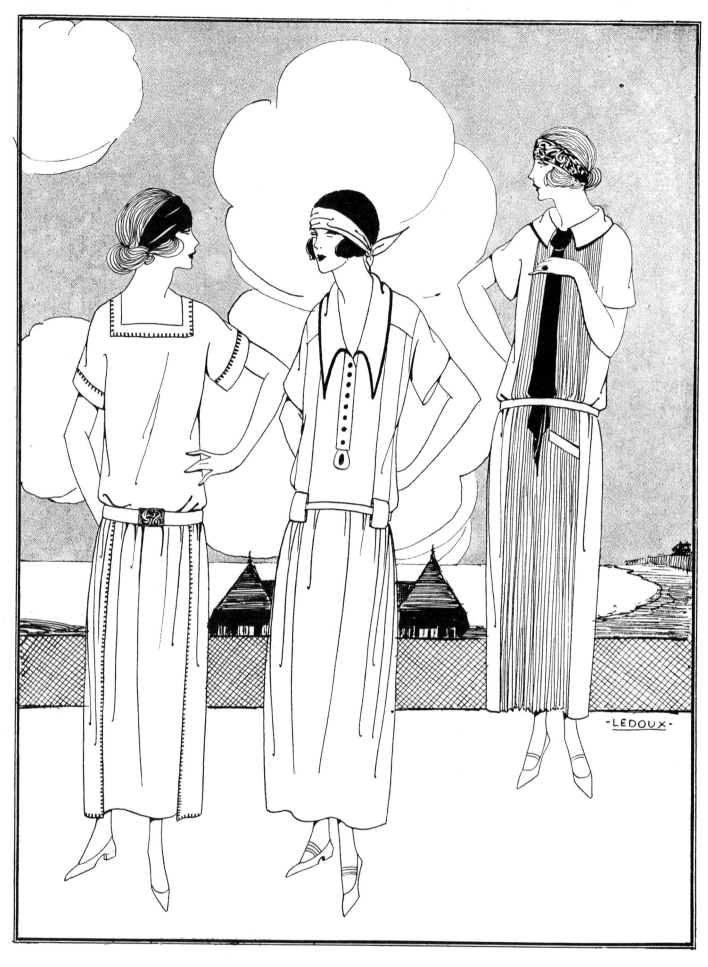

Robe de serge blanche, brodée
de points de soie rouge vif.

Robe en toile blanche
formant chemisier.

Robe en jersey de laine blanc; cravate de satin
noir. Jupe et corsage plissés en panneaux.

White serge ; bright red
silk points embroidered.

White cloth shirtwaist
dress.

White wool jersey, black satin tie.
Pleated skirt and bodice.

AT THE DEAUVILLE SPORTING CLUB

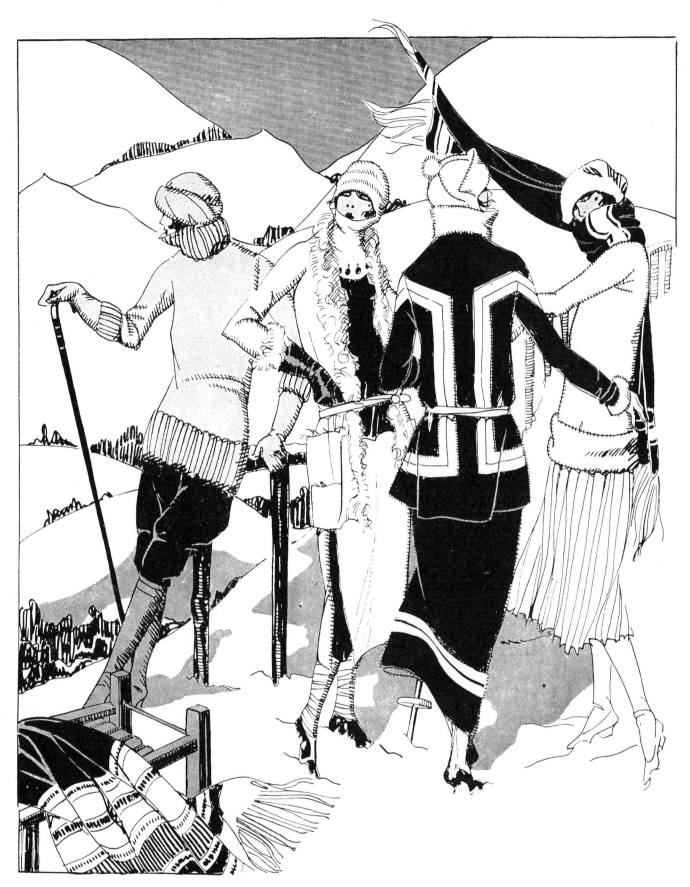

Turban en Kashavella blond drapé; chandail en tricot du ton. Culotte de peau «capucin» et bottines en cuir assorti.

Blond Kashavella *turban; matching knitted sweater. Nasturtium leather breeches and matching leather boots.*

Costume de peau mate blanche, doublé de mongolie, ouvert sur un gilet de Crépella double bleu «Madone» qui se retrouve en plis creux d'un côté à la jupe. Gants de peau bleu «Madone», doublés de mongolie.

White matte leather, lined with *Mongolian lamb over blue double Crépella waistcoat. Blue leather gloves, lined with Mongolian lamb.*

Costume en Velursine rouge laqué, brodé de soie blanche et garni de lapin blanc.

Lacquer red Velursine, *embroidered with white silk and trimmed with white rabbit fur.*

Chandail en laine grattée blanche s'assortissant au béret; jupe en flanelle plissée. Echarpe en Kashavella «corail», drapée blanc.

White wool sweater. Pleated *flannel skirt. Coral Kashavella scarf, white stripe.*

OR DO YOU PREFER SNOW?

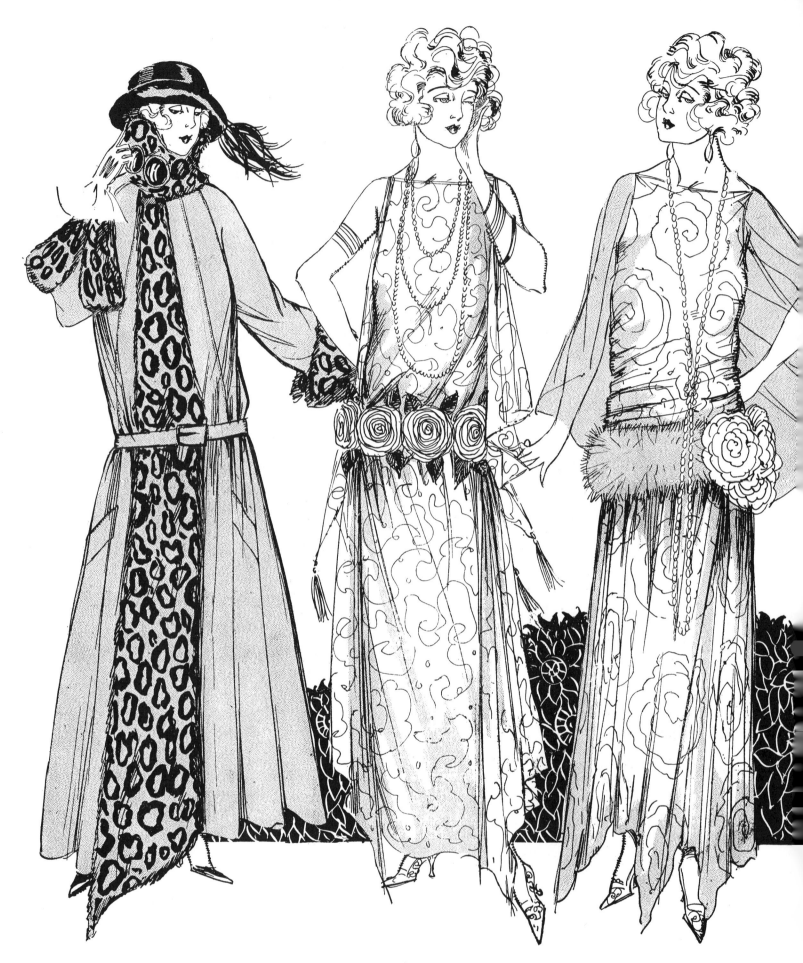

Manteau à deux fins et reversible en peau blanche, garni de chat tigré ; intérieur en velours gris.

White leather coat trimmed with spotted cat, reversible to grey velvet.

Robe que portera Mlle Sorel dans La Mégère apprivoisée, *en tissu lamé «or» et ceinture de roses.*

Gown Mlle. Sorel will wear in La Mégère apprivoisée [The Taming of the Shrew], of gold lamé with a belt of roses.

Robe en dentelle de soie mauve ; ceinture de renard gris et pouf de fleurs.

Gown of mauve silk lace, grey fox waistband and flower pouf.

Mademoiselle Cécile Sorel has left for America. There she will represent

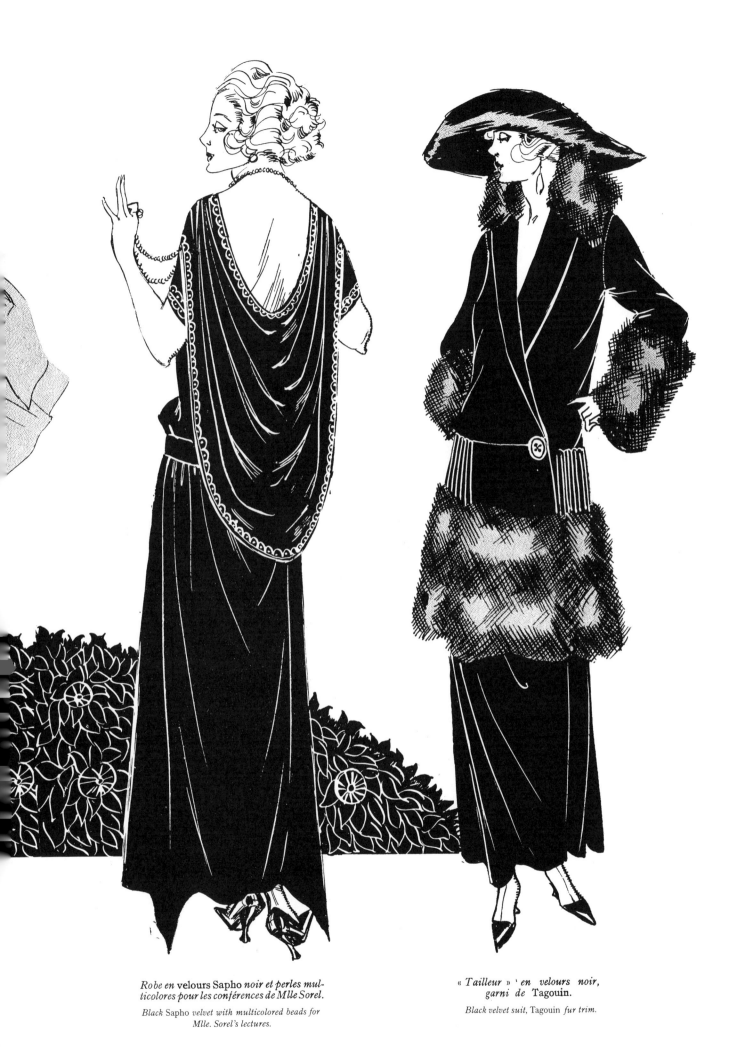

Robe en **velours** *Sapho noir et perles mul-*
ticolores pour les conférences de Mlle Sorel.

Black Sapho *velvet with multicolored beads for*
Mlle. Sorel's lectures.

« Tailleur » ' en velours noir,
garni de Tagouin.

Black velvet suit, Tagouin fur trim.

French art and good taste with these costumes from D O U C E T.

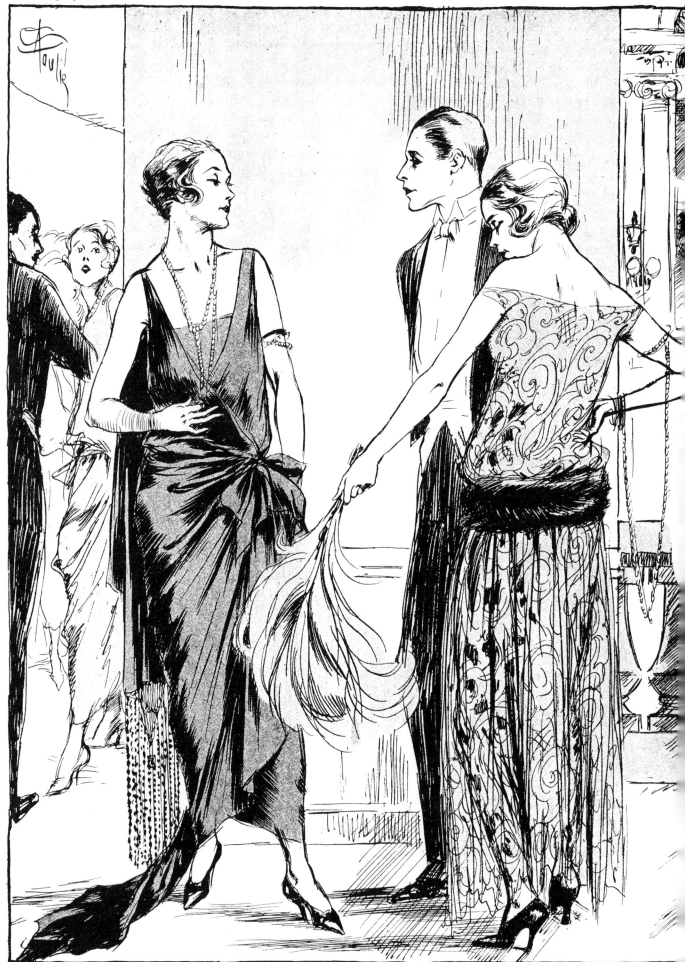

*Robe en velours
Sapho noir. Frange
de diamants et rubis.*

*Black Sapho velvet.
Diamonds and rubis
fringe.*

WORTH

*Robe de dentelle d'or;
ceinture de vison.*

*Golden lace; mink
belt.*

MOLYNEUX

*Fourreau de jais sur
satin noir.*

*Jet sheath over black
satin.*

DOUCET

WORTH   MOLYNEUX

A SUBSCRIPTION

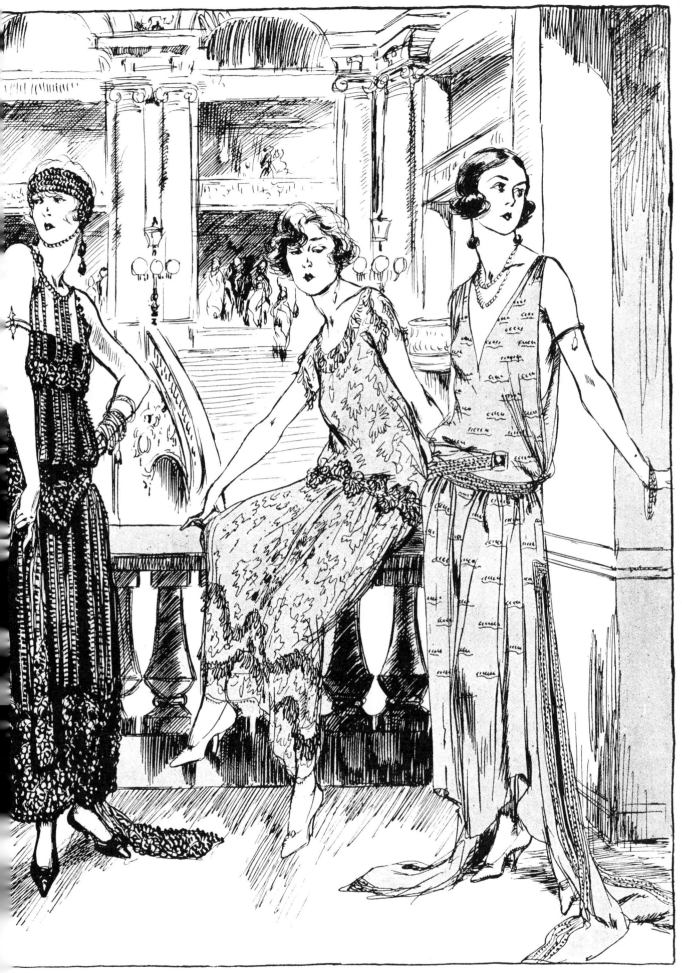

Robe de dentelle lamée «argent», garnie de ruban lamé.

Silver lace.

DŒUILLET

(d'après Photo Rahma)

Robe en lamé «turquoise», brodée de diamants.

Turquoise coloured lamé, rhinestone embroidery.

RENÉE

DOUCET   DŒUILLET   RENEE

NIGHT AT THE OPERA

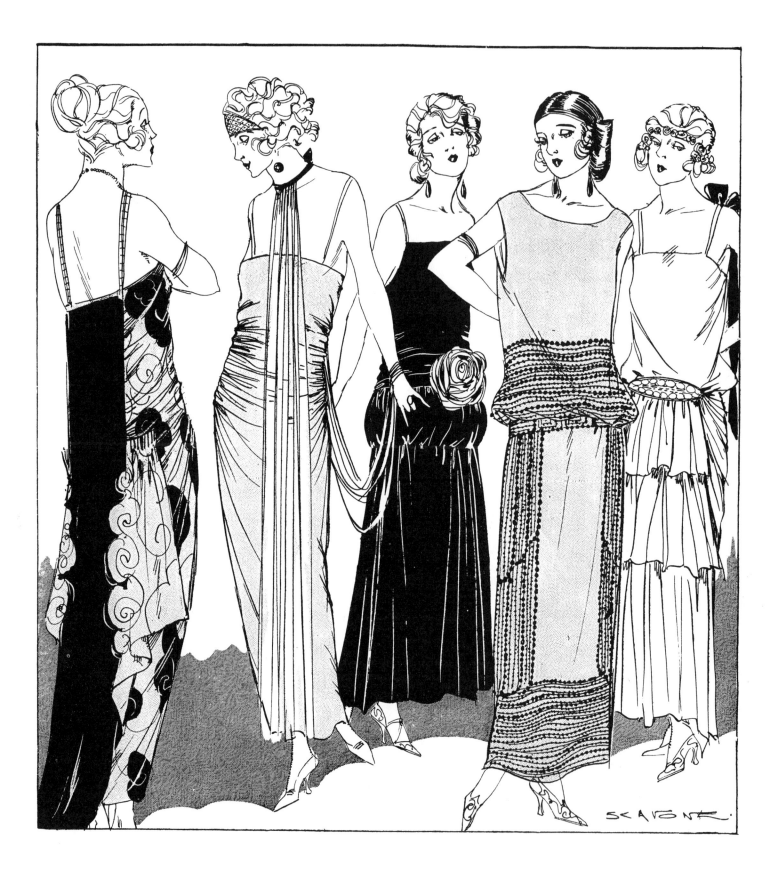

Robe en Sardanapale *or,* *noir et rouge ancien.*	Robe de style en velours Frisson « vert Empire ».	Robe en velours Sapho lamé rouge.	Robe de crêpe Athénien blond, garnie de perles.	Robe en crêpe Nizam *mauve ; nœud et pans en velours violet sur l'épaule gauche.*
Golden, black and antique red Sardanapale.	*"Empire" green silk frisson velvet.*	*Red lamé* Sapho *velvet.*	*Blond* Athenian crêpe, *beaded trim.*	*Mauve* Nizam *crêpe; violet velvet bow and streamers on left shoulder.*
DOUCET	**CALLOT Sœurs**	**WORTH**	**PREMET**	**WORTH**

AT THE BAL
DE LA
COUTURE
(December 8)

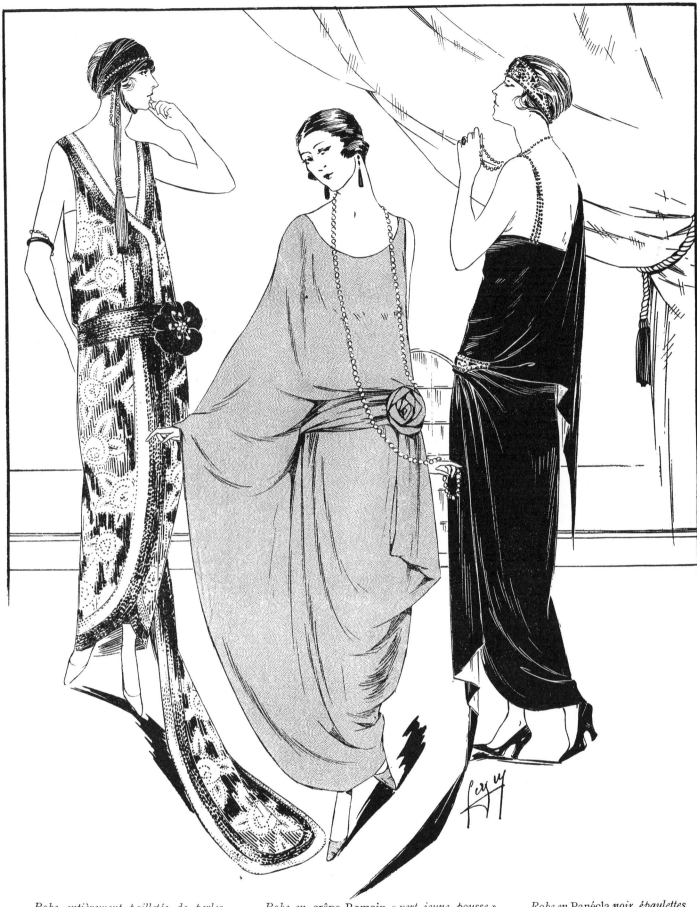

*Robe entièrement pailletée de perles,
de tubes de cristal et de jais ;
fleur de célophane à la ceinture.*

Pearl beads, bugle beads of
crystal and jet; cellophane
flower at waist.

MOLYNEUX

Robe en crêpe Romain « *vert jeune pousse* »,
*drapée sous une grosse fleur. Un bras est nu,
l'autre enveloppé par le drapé même de la robe.*

Sprout green crêpe Romain, *draped from a
large flower. One arm is bare, the other
enveloped by the drape of the dress itself.*

Jean PATOU

Robe en Panécla *noir, épaulettes
de strass ; diadème et agrafe
de côté en strass et onyx.*

Black Panécla, *rhinestone shoulder
straps; rhinestone and onyx headband
and clasp.*

MOLYNEUX

SOME GOWNS SEEN ON CHRISTMAS EVE

(Creations by Molyneux and Jean Patou)

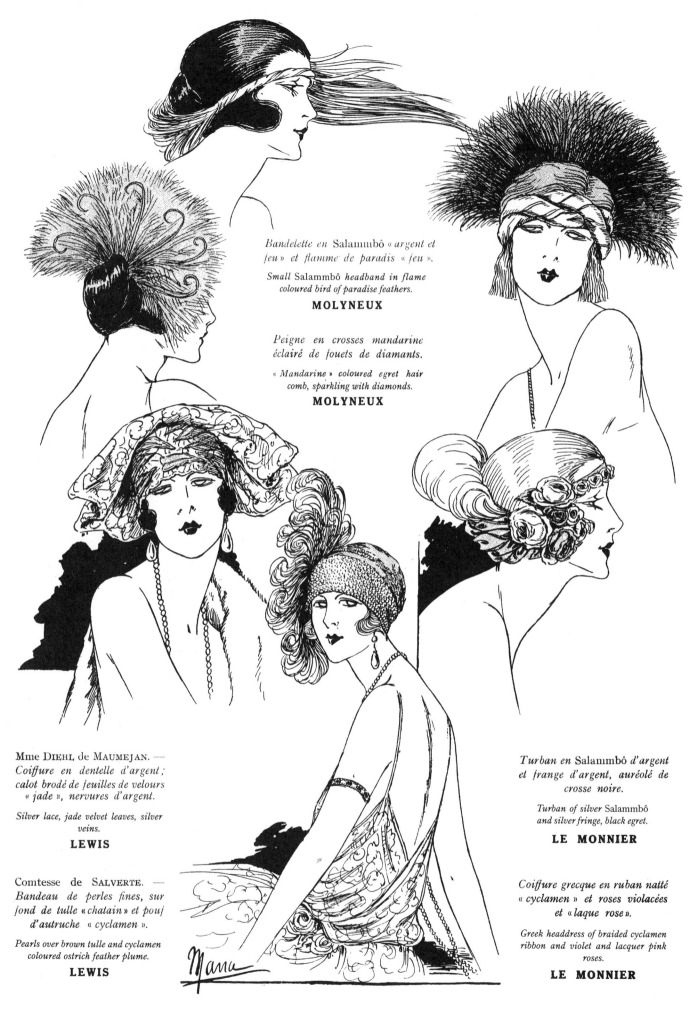

Bandelette en Salammbô « argent et feu » et flamme de paradis « feu ».

Small Salammbô headband in flame coloured bird of paradise feathers.

MOLYNEUX

Peigne en crosses mandarine éclairé de fouets de diamants.

« Mandarine » coloured egret hair comb, sparkling with diamonds.

MOLYNEUX

Mme DIEHL de MAUMEJAN. — *Coiffure en dentelle d'argent ; calot brodé de feuilles de velours « jade », nervures d'argent.*

Silver lace, jade velvet leaves, silver veins.

LEWIS

Comtesse de SALVERTE. — *Bandeau de perles fines, sur fond de tulle « chatain » et pouf d'autruche « cyclamen ».*

Pearls over brown tulle and cyclamen coloured ostrich feather plume.

LEWIS

Turban en Salammbô d'argent et frange d'argent, auréolé de crosse noire.

Turban of silver Salammbô and silver fringe, black egret.

LE MONNIER

Coiffure grecque en ruban natté « cyclamen » et roses violacées et « laque rose ».

Greek headdress of braided cyclamen ribbon and violet and lacquer pink roses.

LE MONNIER

A FEW PRETTY HEADDRESSES NOTED AT THE BAL DES PETITS LITS BLANCS

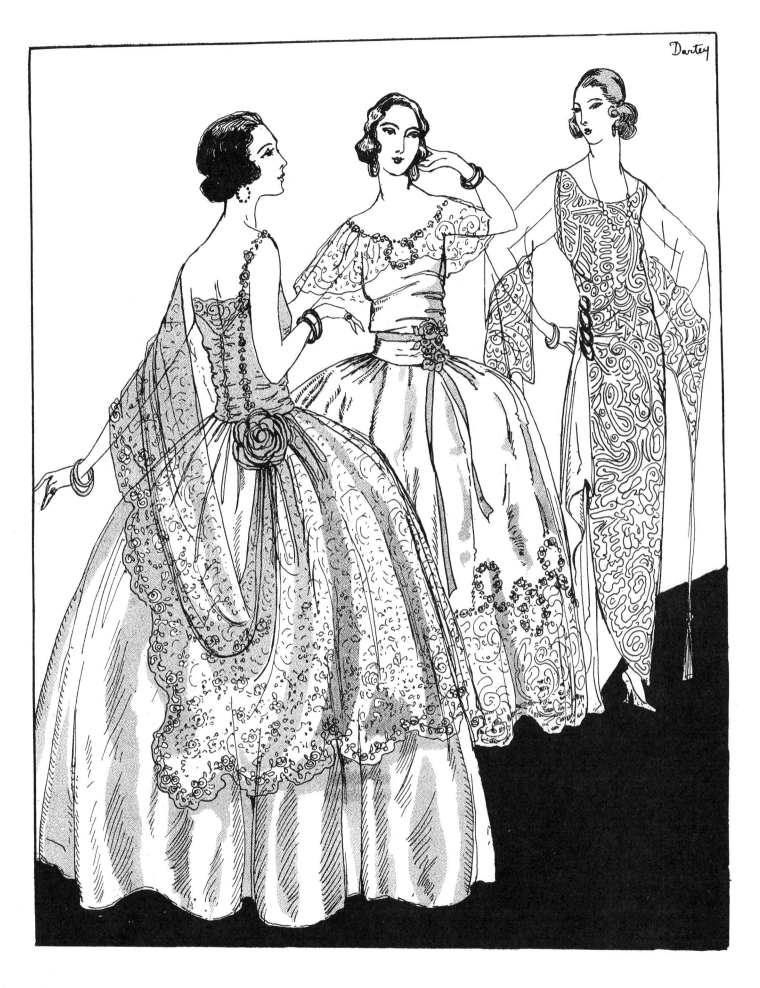

Dartey

Robe en taf-
fetas bleu et
dentelle.

Blue taffeta
and lace.

Robe en faille
« paille » et dentelle
d'argent.

Straw coloured faille
and silver lace.

Robe en crêpe
« ivoire » et crêpe
brodé or.

Ivory coloured crêpe,
golden embroidery.

CHEZ
LUCILE
11, Rue de Penthièvre

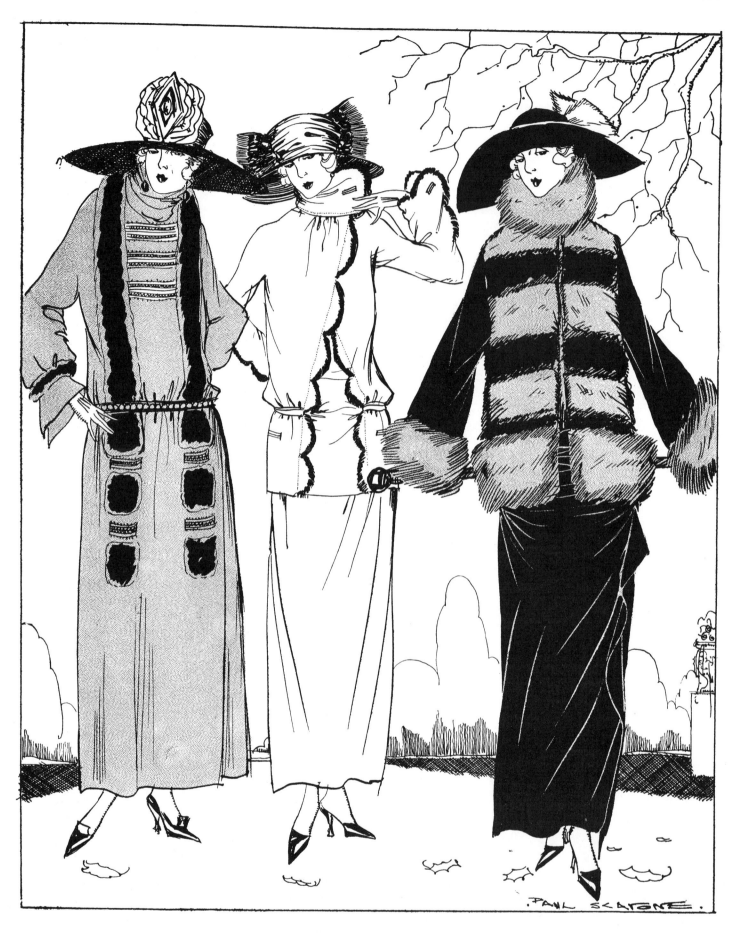

Manteau en Velur-
sine « vert-de-gris »,
garni de loutre.

Verdigris coloured
Velursine ; otter fur
trimming.

« Tailleur » en Perllaine
« perle », bordée de pe-
tites bandes de fourrure.

Pearl coloured Perl-
laine; edged with narrow
fur bands.

Veste de fourrure noire
et blanche ; manches et
robe de velours Sapho.

Black and white fur ;
Sapho velvet gown
and sleeves.

WINTER ISN'T OVER

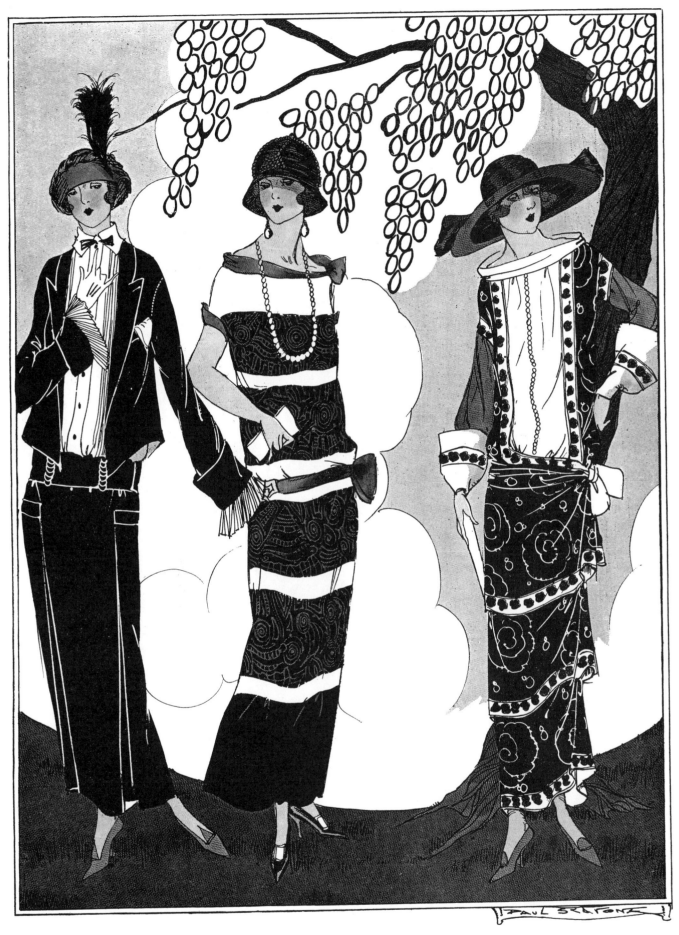

Robe-tailleur en Crépella;
blouse-tailleur en linon blanc.

Crepélla tailored ensemble;
white linen tailored blouse.

Robe en foulard im-
primé, uni et blanc.

Printed, plain and
white foulard.

Robe en foulard, Organ-
dina et galons à fleurs.

Foulard, Organdina and
flowered braid.

TAILORED ENSEMBLE AND DRESSES OF FOULARD

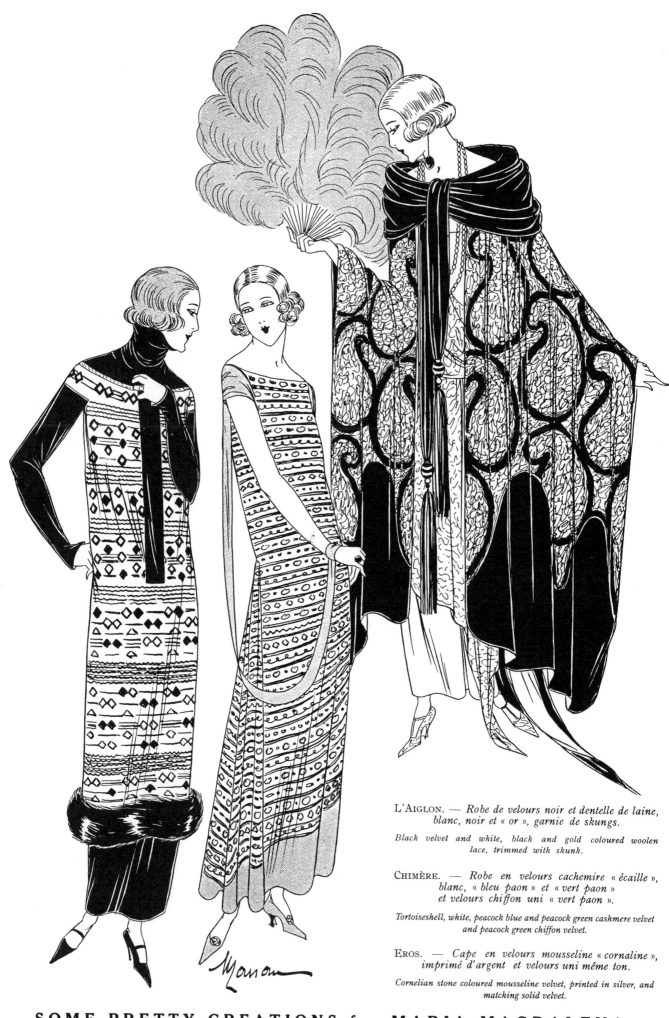

L'AIGLON. — *Robe de velours noir et dentelle de laine, blanc, noir et « or », garnie de skungs.*

Black velvet and white, black and gold coloured woolen lace, trimmed with skunk.

CHIMÈRE. — *Robe en velours cachemire « écaille », blanc, « bleu paon » et « vert paon » et velours chiffon uni « vert paon ».*

Tortoiseshell, white, peacock blue and peacock green cashmere velvet and peacock green chiffon velvet.

EROS. — *Cape en velours mousseline « cornaline », imprimé d'argent et velours uni même ton.*

Cornelian stone coloured mousseline velvet, printed in silver, and matching solid velvet.

SOME PRETTY CREATIONS from MARIA-MAGDALENA
10, Rue du Commandant-Marchand

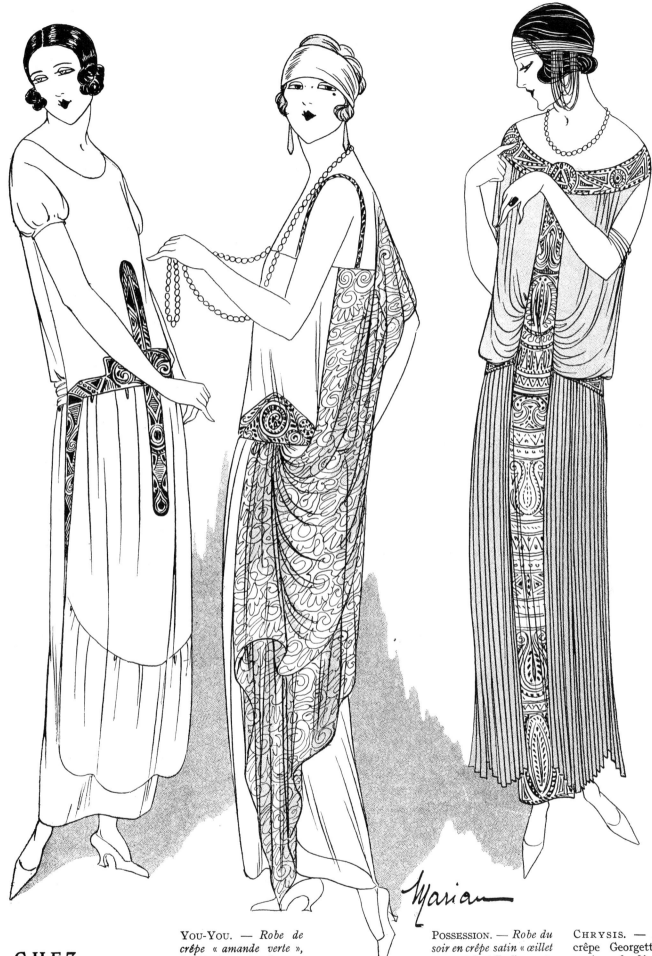

CHEZ
CAUËT
6, Rue de la Paix, 6

YOU-YOU. — *Robe de crêpe « amande verte », brodée de perles de tons cachemire.*

Almond coloured crêpe; cashmere shawl—coloured bead embroidery.

POSSESSION. — *Robe du soir en crêpe satin « œillet rose » et dentelle d'or mat ; motif perlé de strass et argent sur velours du ton.*

Pink satin crêpe and matte gold lace; rhinestone and silver beaded ornament over matching velvet.

CHRYSIS. — *Robe de crêpe Georgette « turquoise », brodée de perles et paillettes de tons changeants.*

Turquoise crêpe Georgette, embroidered with iridescent beads and paillettes.

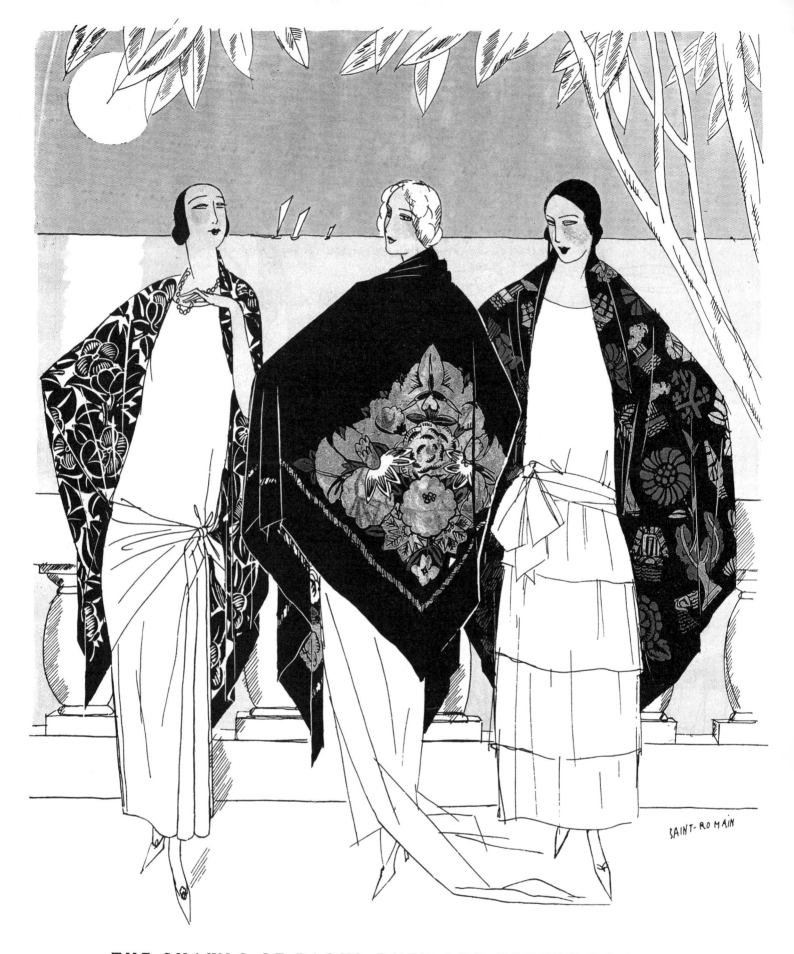

SAINT-ROMAIN

THE SHAWLS OF RAOUL DUFY AND ROBERT BONFILS

PRODUCED BY

BIANCHINI, FÉRIER.

*To our great regret, we are unable to convey in these drawings the richness
and variety of colour of these ravishing shawls.*

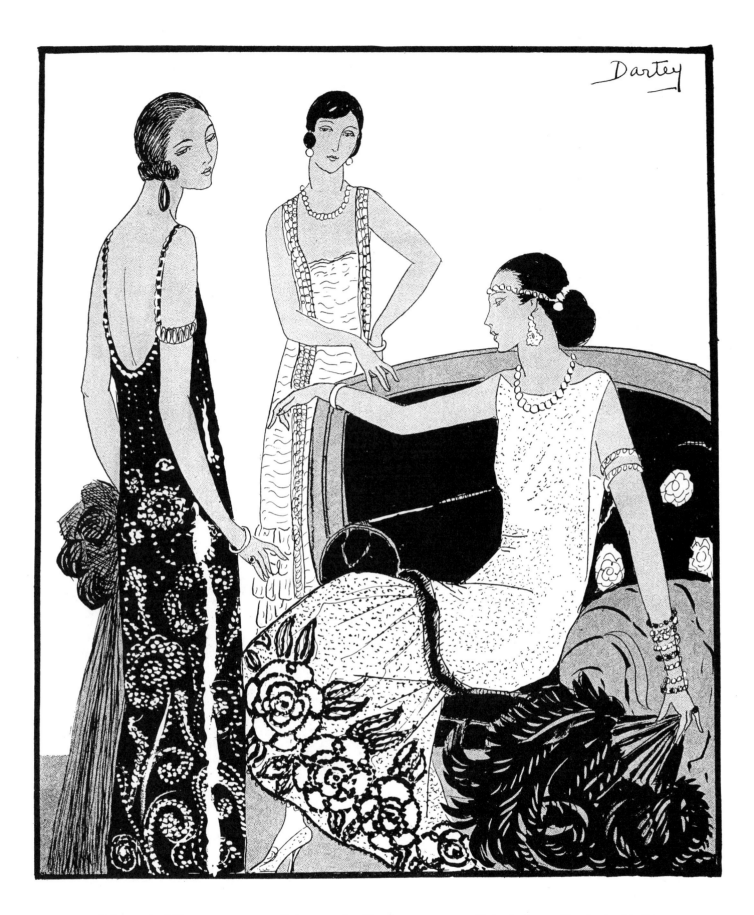

*Robe en crêpe Minerve
noir brodé « or ».*

*Robe en moire Mystère
souple « bleu saphir »;
broderies « argent ».*

*Robe de panne blanche, brodée d'un
semis de perles d'or ; broderies d'or.*

■   ■   ■

*Black Minerve crêpe,
gold embroidery.*

*« Sapphire blue » coloured,
Mystère moire, silver embroidery.*

*White panné velvet, scattered gold
beads; gold embroidery.*

A PARTY AT THE CHÂTEAU

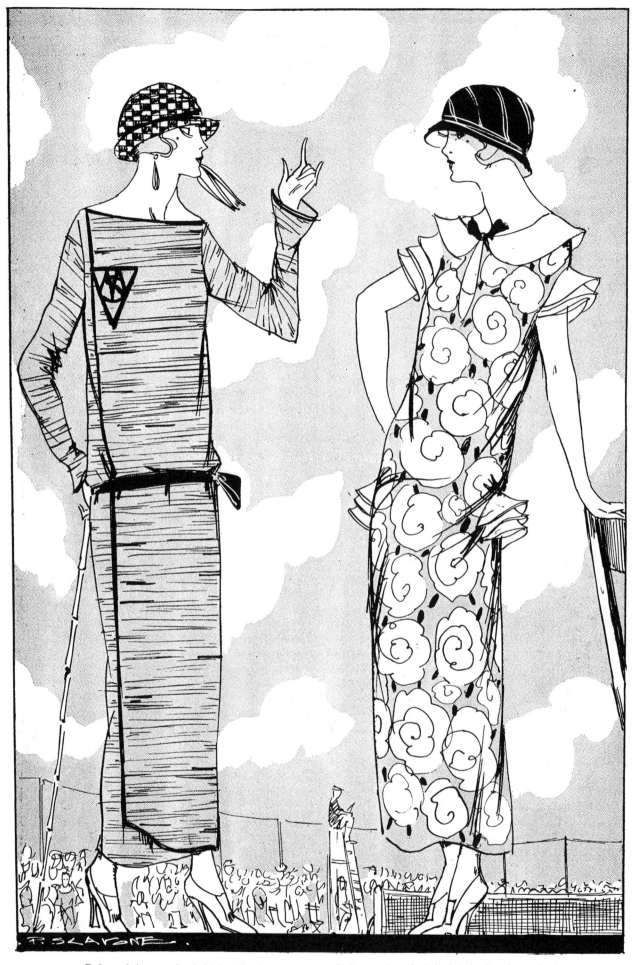

*Robe en lainage gris ; initiale et bordure
en cuir noir.*

Grey wool; black leather piping and monogram.

*Robe en tissu imprimé à fond noir ; volants
d'organdi blanc.*

Print on black ground; white organdy flounces.

AT THE DEAUVILLE SPORTING CLUB
(DAVIS CUP)

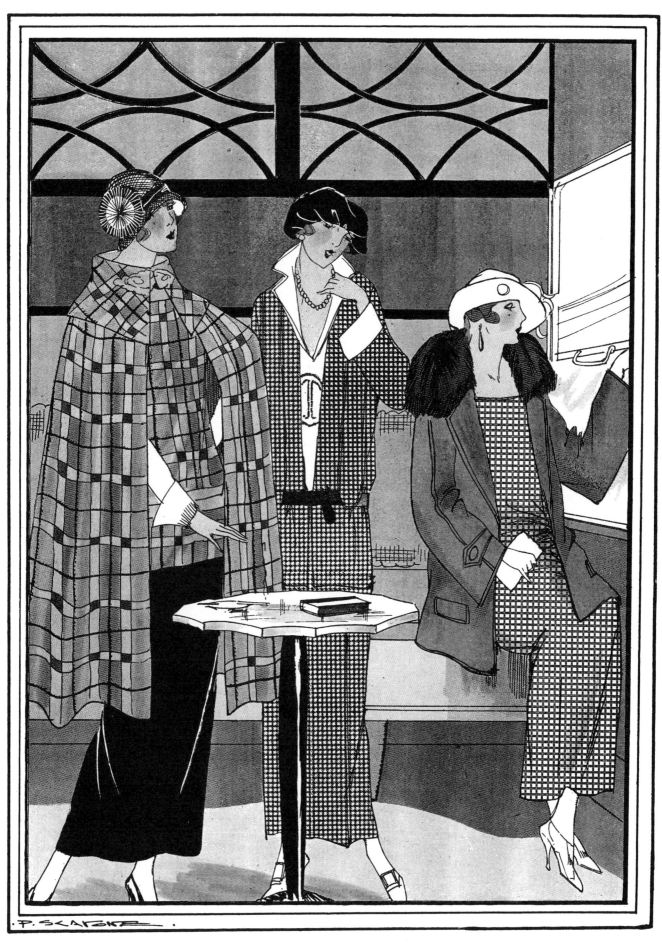

. P. SCAFONE .

Robe et cape de voyage
« écossais »; lainage uni:

Plaid wool
dress and cape.

Tailleur à damier et ceinture en peau;
parements et col en Organdina blanc.

Checkered suit and leather belt, with
Organdina cuffs and collar.

Veste en peau de Suède rouge;
robe en lainage tissé du ton.

Red suede jacket; matching wool
dress.

ON THE TRAIN BLEU

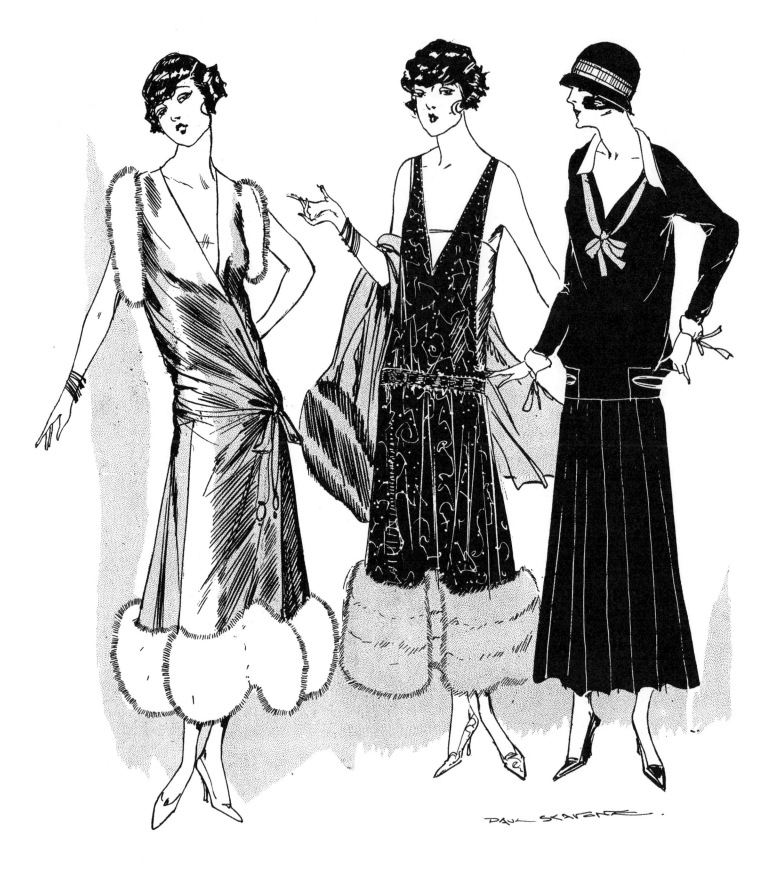

Déshabillé en crêpe satin « ibis », garni de cygne.

Déshabillé of ibis coloured satin crêpe, trimmed with swansdown.

Robe du soir « émeraude », perlée de cristal et ourlée de marabout du ton.

Emerald coloured crystal beads, trimmed with matching marabou.

Robe-tailleur en reps marine, éclairée de biais « amande ».

Navy blue rep, with almond green coloured bias trim.

AT THE THÉÂTRE ANTOINE
THE OUTFITS OF Mlle. GABY MORLAY
CREATIONS BY JEAN PATOU

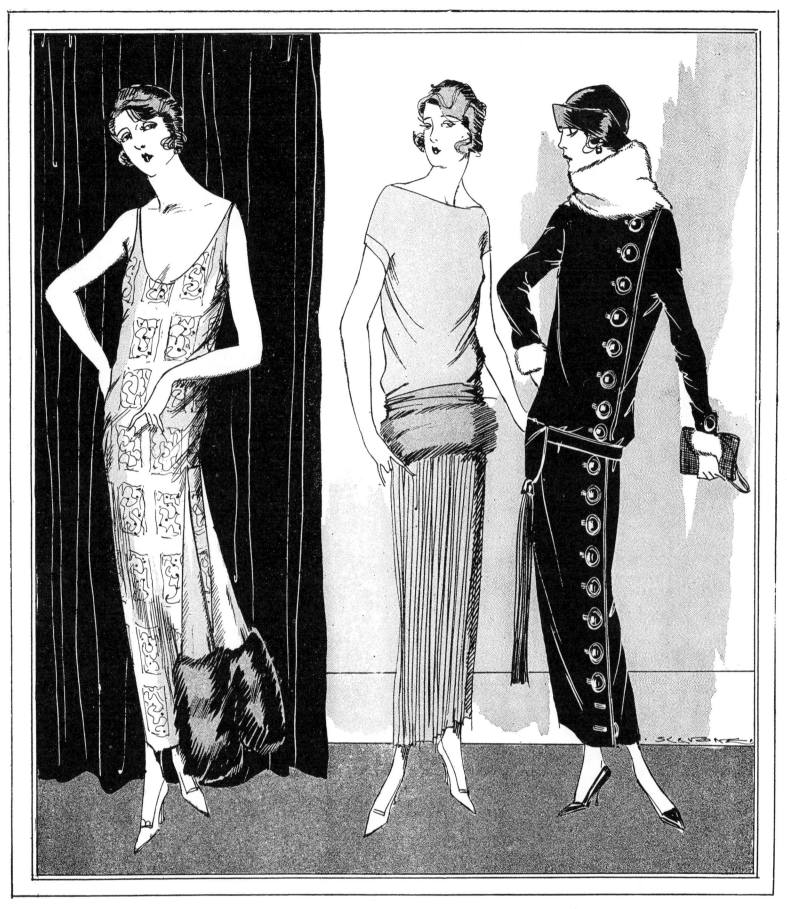

Robe du soir en lamé argent «cyclamen» quadrillée de perles fines et de cristal, garnie de renard bleu.

Cyclamen coloured silver lamé checkered with pearls and crystal, trimmed with blue fox.

Robe en crêpe Marocain « grège », *ourlé de renard même teinte.*

Greige crêpe Marocain *trimmed with matching fox.*

Robe de crêpe Romain *noir bordée de cuir noir; poche avec grand gland.*

Black Roman crêpe, *edged with black kid; pocket with long tassel.*

THE TOILETTES OF Mlle. YVONNE DE BRAY IN THE TRIUMPHANT REVIVAL OF
LA FEMME NUE [THE NUDE WOMAN] AT THE VAUDEVILLE ARE CREATIONS OF

DRECOLL

136, Avenue des Champs-Élysées.

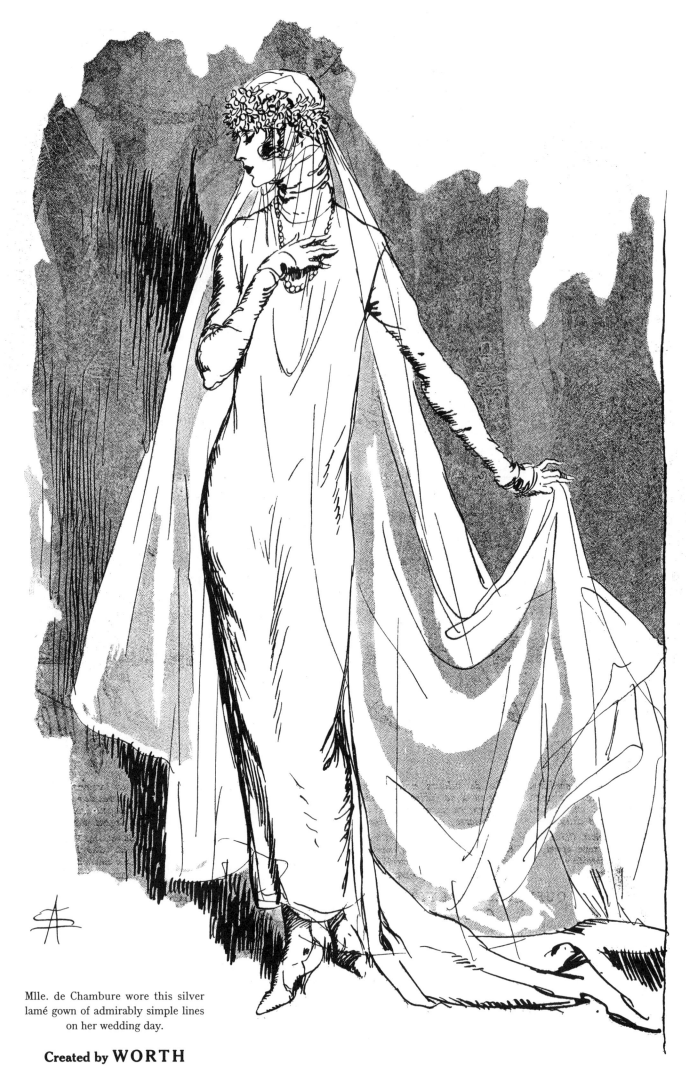

Mlle. de Chambure wore this silver
lamé gown of admirably simple lines
on her wedding day.

Created by WORTH

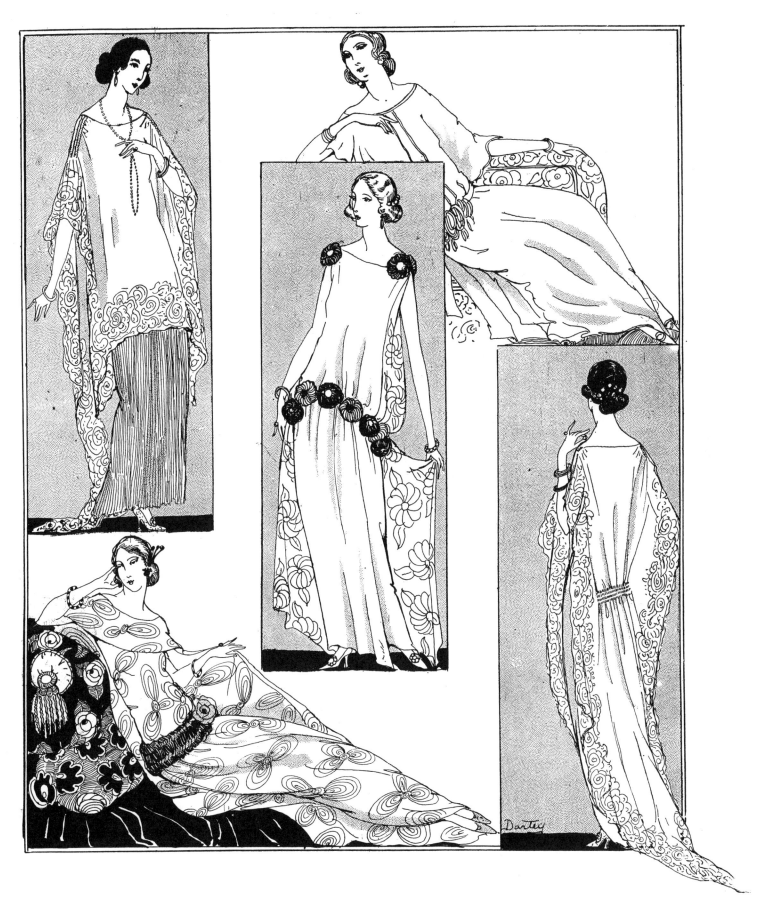

Déshabillé en crêpe Romain « *rouge ancien* » *et dentelle de soie rouge.*

Antique red Roman crêpe *and red silk lace.*

Robe d'intérieur en crêpe Javanais *bleu* « *jade* », *garni de biais de crêpe.*

Jade blue Javanese crêpe, *trimmed with bias crêpe piping.*

Robe d'intérieur en crêpe Athénien *et broché jaune* « *citron* »; *fleurs de laine noires et jaunes.*

Plain Athenian crêpe *and lemon coloured yellow brocade; black and yellow woolen flowers.*

Robe d'intérieur en crêpe Korrigan « *bleu Nattier* » *broché; ceinture de fourrure; rose rouge.*

Nattier blue brocaded Korrigan crêpe; *fur belt; red rose.*

Déshabillé en crêpe Romain « *brique* »; *dentelle de soie.*

Brick coloured Roman crêpe; *silk lace.*

FOR THE INTIMACY OF THE HOME
CREATIONS FROM DOUCET

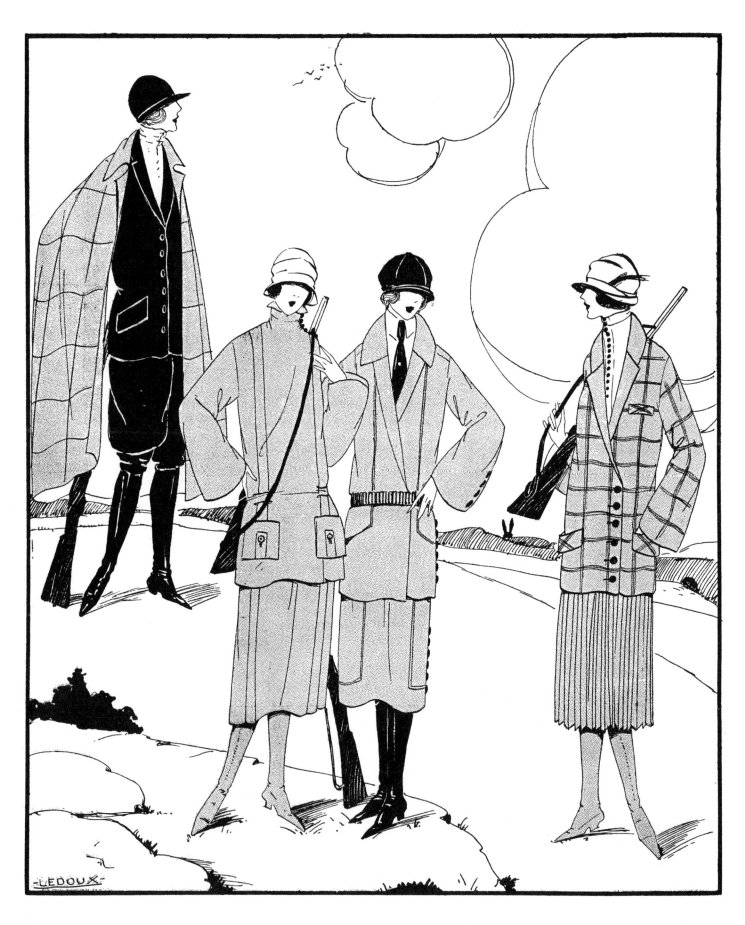

Cape en Kasha quadrillé *sur costume de velours* van Dyck « nègre ».

Costume de chasse en Buracotta « castor ».

Costume en Mouflavella vert sombre, *garni de boutons noirs.*

Costume en Duvetine quadrillée. *Jupe plissée.*

■   ■   ■   ■

Checked Kasha *cape, over a brown* Van Dyke velvet *costume.*

Beaver coloured Buracotta *hunting costume.*

Dark green Mouflavella; *trimmed with black buttons.*

Checkered Duvetine. *Pleated skirt.*

FOR THE HUNT

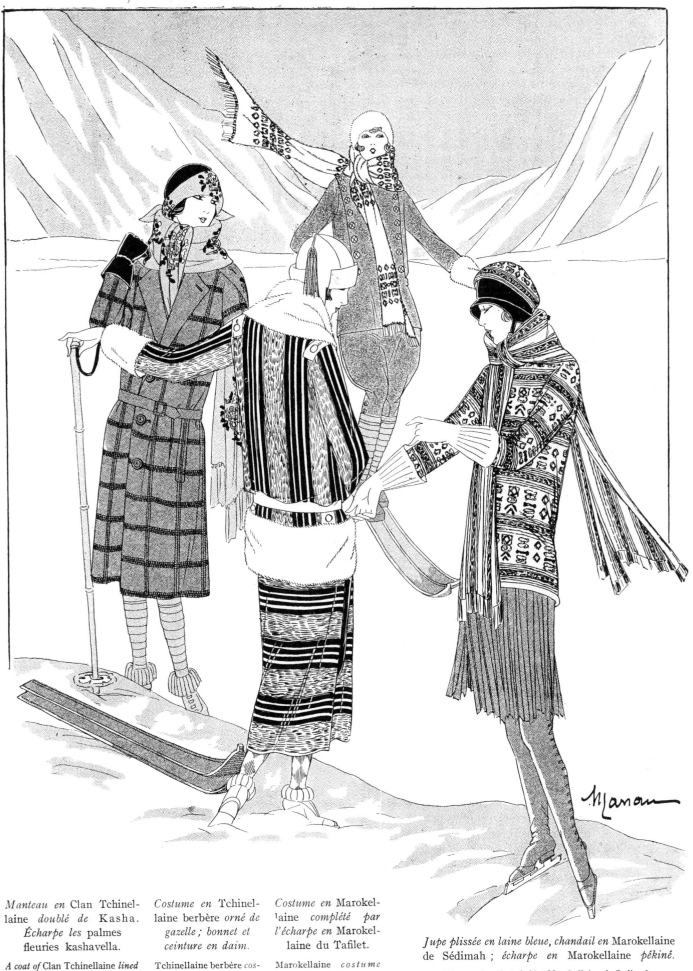

Manteau en Clan Tchinellaine *doublé de* Kasha. *Écharpe* les palmes fleuries kashavella.

A coat of Clan Tchinellaine *lined with* Kasha. *«Les palmes fleuries»* Kashasvella *scarf.*

Costume en Tchinellaine berbère *orné de gazelle ;* bonnet et ceinture en daim.

Tchinellaine berbère *costume trimmed with gazelle fur, deerskin cap and belt.*

Costume en Marokellaine *complété par l'écharpe en* Marokellaine du Tafilet.

Marokellaine *costume with* Marokellaine du Tafilet *scarf.*

Jupe plissée en laine bleue, chandail en Marokellaine de Sédimah ; *écharpe en* Marokellaine *pékiné.*

Blue woolen pleated skirt, Marokellaine de Sedimah *sweater and* Marokellaine pekiné *scarf.*

FABRICS BY RODIER

ARE YOU GOING TO CHAMONIX FOR THE OLYMPICS?

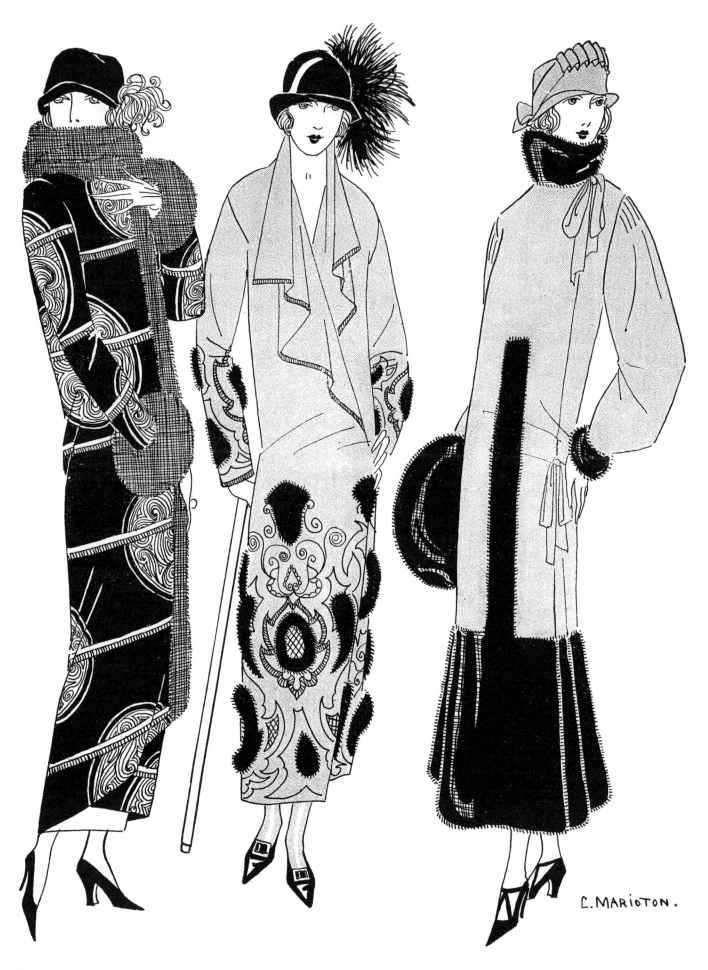

C. MARIOTON.

Manteau en Fulgurante *noire brodée argent et noir, bordé de renard gris.*

Black Fulgurante, *silver and black embroidered edged with grey fox fur.*

Manteau en Drapella « *rouge éteint* ». *Motifs en castor et en broderies rouges.*

Antique red Drapella, *beaver fur and red embroidery.*

Manteau en Duvetine «*vert sombre*» *garni de loutre en forme dans le bas.*

Dark green Duvetine *trimmed with otter at hem.*

COATS FOR MILDER DAYS

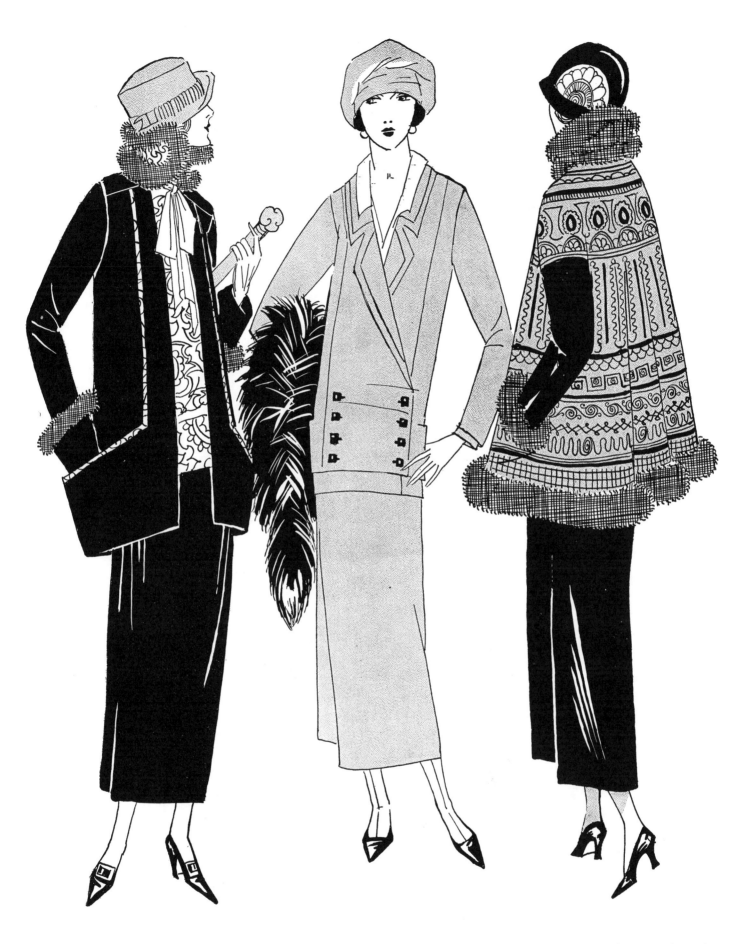

*Tailleur en velours de laine «marine», s'ouvrant
sur un gilet de velours blanc brodé bleu.*

Navy blue woolen velvet, white
velvet waistcoat, blue embroidery.

*Tailleur en reps «aubergine»
bordé de daim plus clair.*

Aubergine coloured rep, edged with
lighter deerskin.

*Tailleur en Kasha noir et Kasha gris
brodé noir et bleu, garni de petit-gris.*

Black Kasha, and grey Kasha, black and blue
embroidery, trimmed with Siberian squirrel.

SUITS

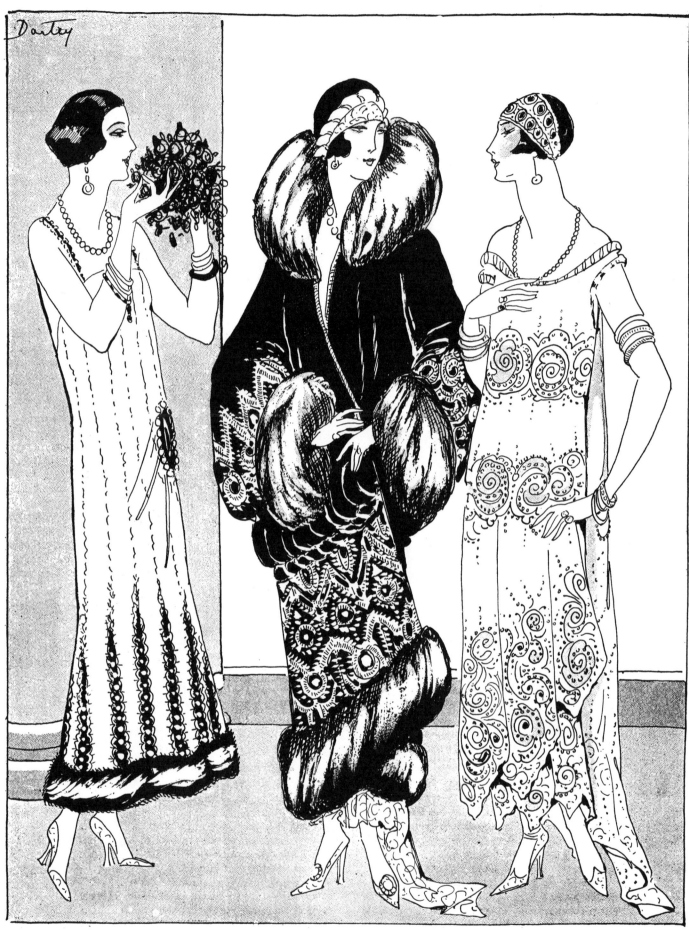

Robe en crêpe Crapote perlée et brodée, légèrement drapée par un motif de bijouterie.

Crapote crêpe *beaded and embroidered draped by a jeweled ornament.*

Manteau en velours Van Dyck « brun » brodé d'or, garni de zibeline.

Brown Van Dyck velvet, *gold embroidered and trimmed with sable.*

Robe en mousseline de soie brodée d'or, jupe enroulée et découpée en pointes.

Chiffon embroidered with gold, *wrapped skirt cut in points.*

A FEW OUTFITS SKETCHED ONE SUNDAY EVENING AT THE RITZ.

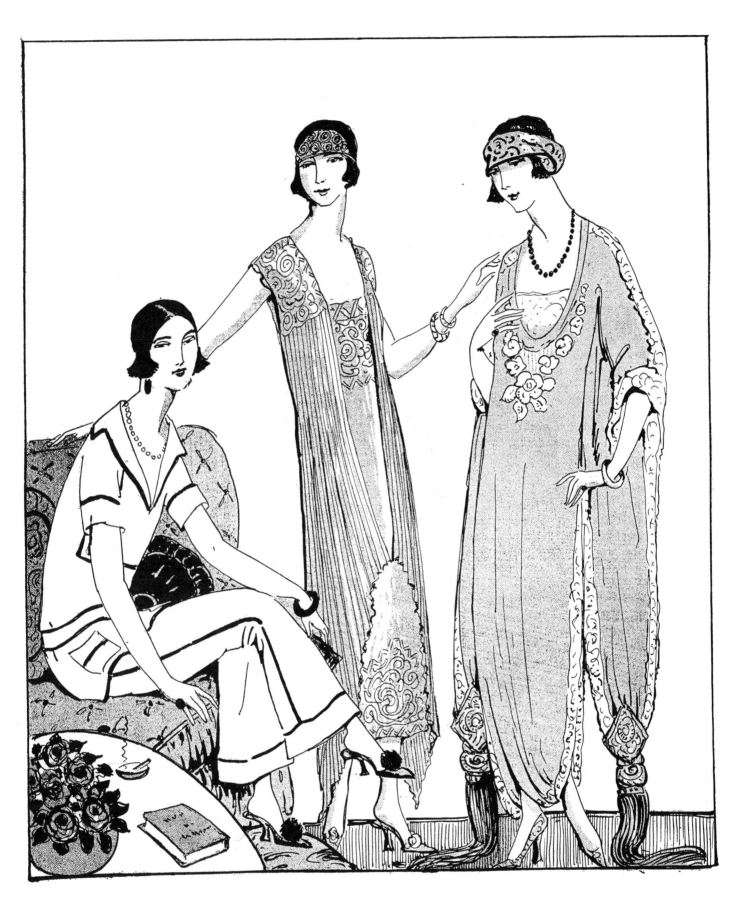

Pyjama en crêpe Crapote
blanc, biais noir.

Pyjamas of white Crapote
crepe and black piping.

MOLYNEUX

*Déshabillé en crêpe de Chine
blanc, dentelle de Milan.*

Déshabillé of white crepe de
Chine and «Milan» lace.

MARTIAL ET ARMAND

Déshabillé en crêpe Georgette
«jade»; dentelle et fleurs d'argent.

Déshabillé of jade coloured crêpe
Georgette, silver lace and flowers.

LUCILE

FOR STAYING HOME

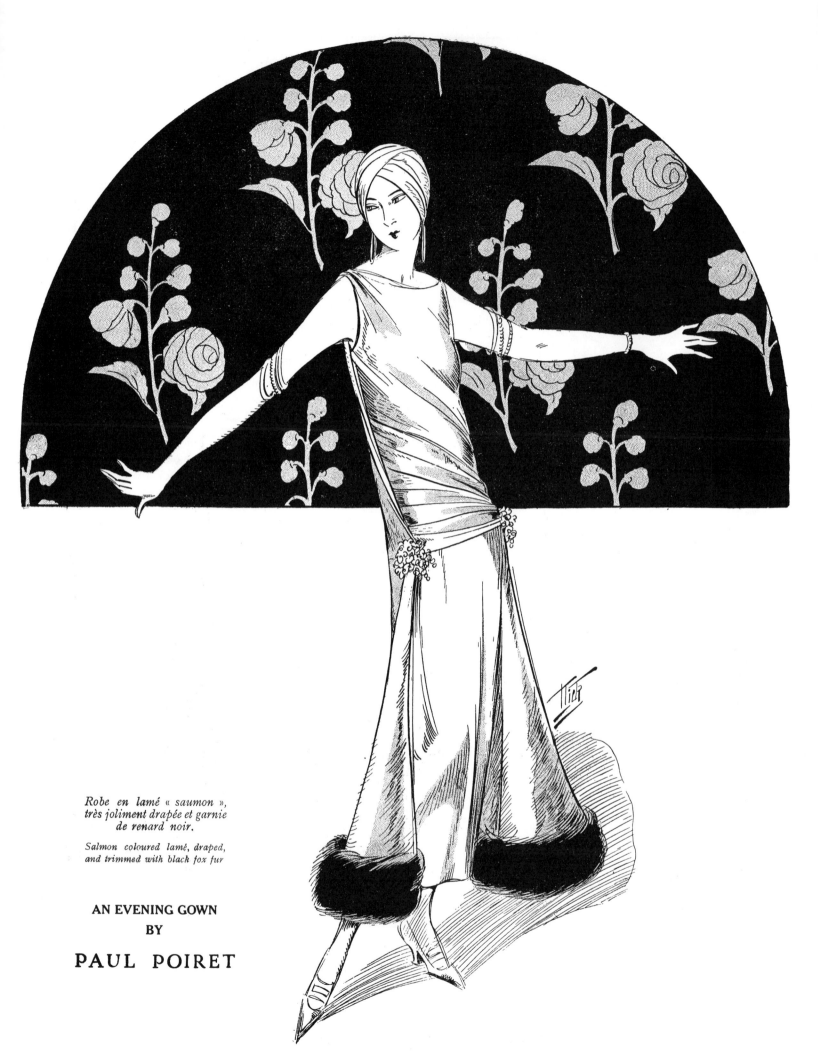

*Robe en lamé « saumon »,
très joliment drapée et garnie
de renard noir.*

*Salmon coloured lamé, draped,
and trimmed with black fox fur*

AN EVENING GOWN
BY

PAUL POIRET

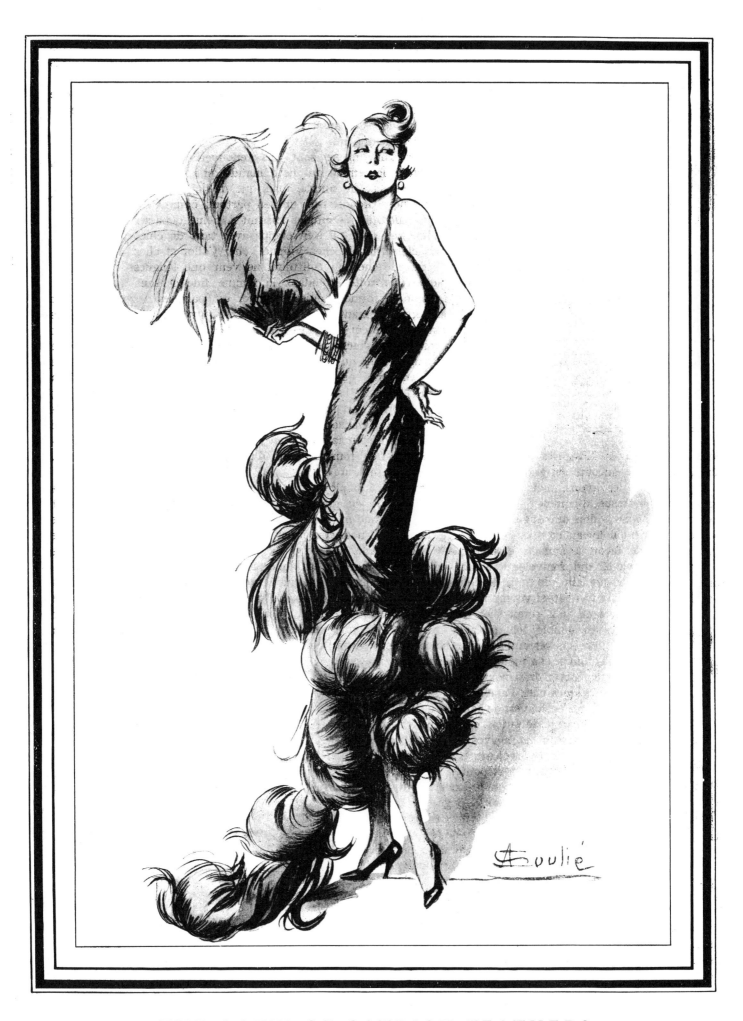

THE GOWN OF OSTRICH FEATHERS

*We are pleased to publish a study that our contributor A.
Soulié has made of the pretty Mme. L——, who consented
to pose in her gown trimmed with ostrich feathers.*

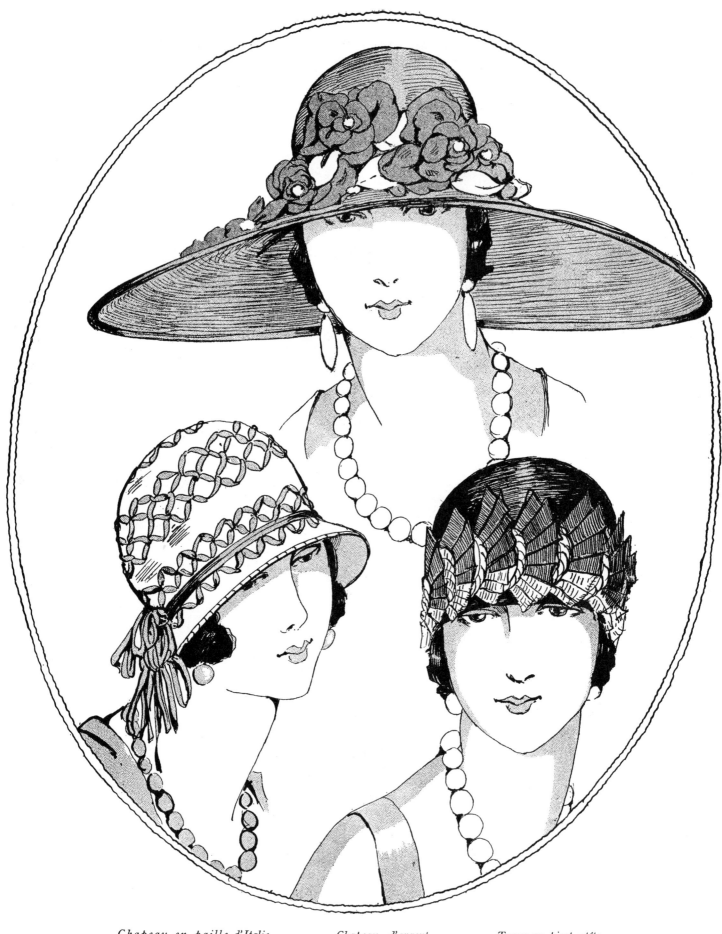

Chapeau en paille d'Italie « géranium », garni de fleurs de velours et de feuilles d'argent.

Geranium coloured Milan straw hat trimmed with velvet flowers and silver leaves.

Chapeau d'argent entrelacs de ruban vert « laitue ».

Silver and lettuce coloured ribbon hat.

Toque en picot « tête-de-nègre », et ruban de faille et d'or.

Tête de nègre coloured hat, and golden faille ribbon.

CHEZ
LUCIE HAMAR

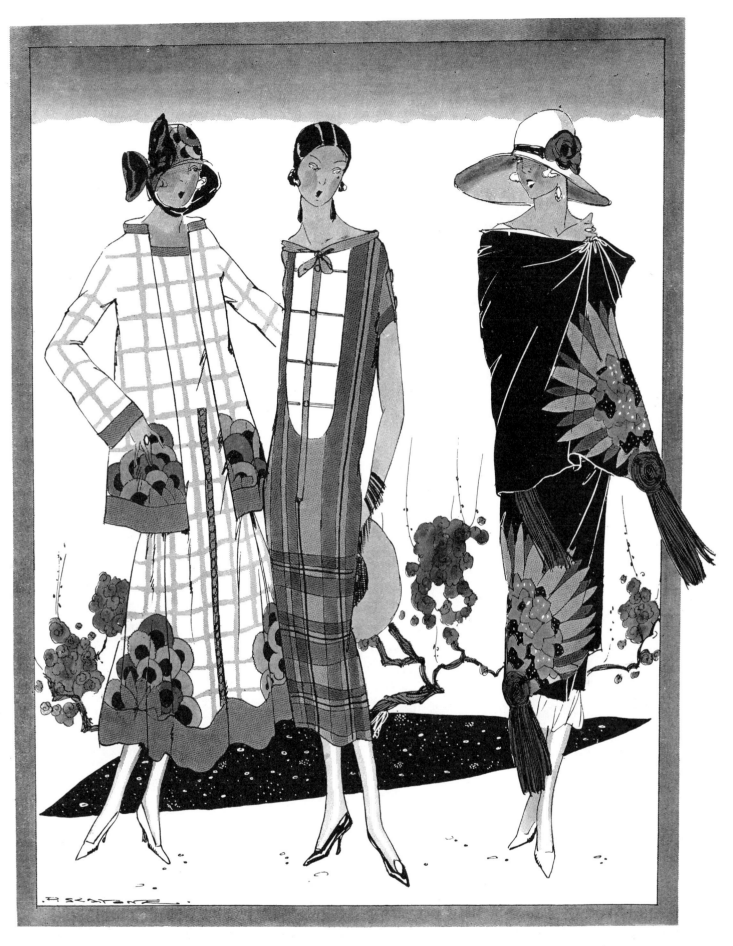

Ensemble de tussor naturel imprimé de fleurs modernes «ambre» et noir sur quadrillé, et bordures « bleu toile ».

Natural tussor printed with amber and black stylized flowers on checkered ground, toile blue borders.

Robe de crêpe Marocain *bleu roy imprimé formant écossais vert et noir par places.*

Printed green and black plaid on blue crêpe Marocain ground.

Châle en crêpe Marocain *noir imprimé, de gros bouquet de rhododendrons jaune orange et bois. Gros glands des mêmes tons.*

Black shawl printed with bouquets of yellow, orange and wood coloured rhododendrons, with long matching tassels.

THESE CREATIONS FROM TISSUS D'ART

8, Rue de Lévis

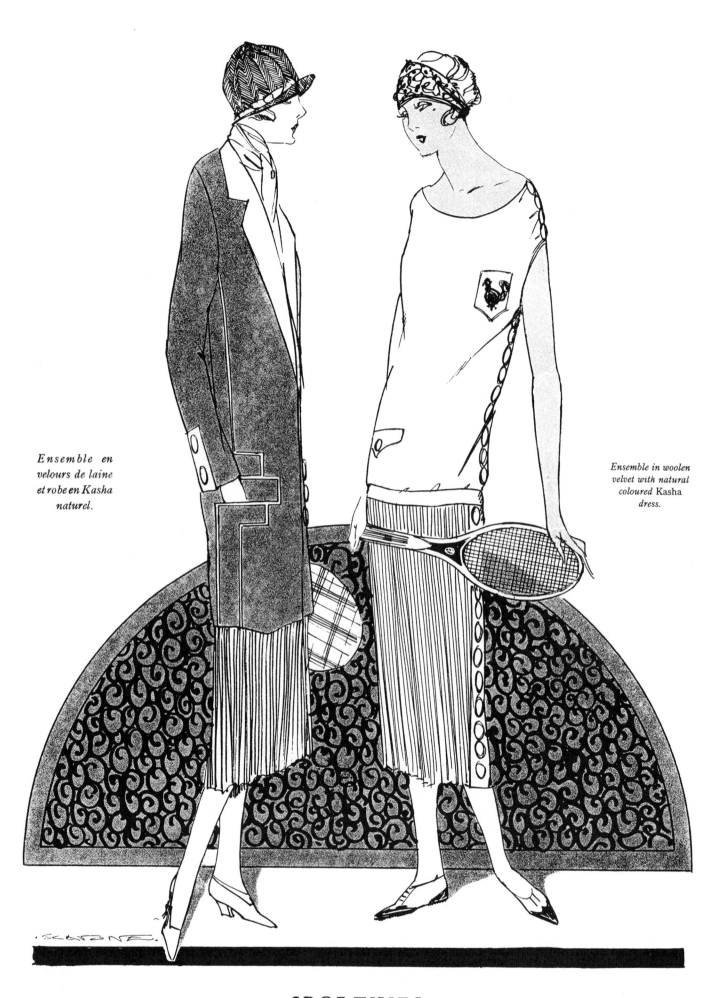

Ensemble en velours de laine et robe en Kasha naturel.

Ensemble in woolen velvet with natural coloured Kasha dress.

SPORTIVES

CRÉATION DE LA SOCIÉTÉ BLANCHE LEBOUVIER
MARIE-LOUISE, Directrice

3, Rue Boudreau

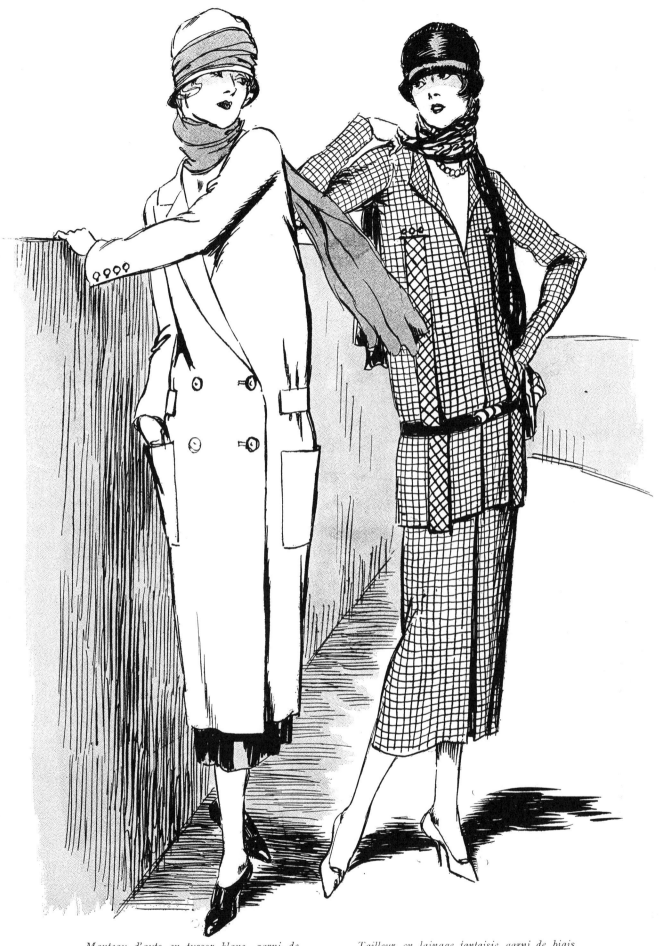

Manteau d'auto en tussor blanc, garni de deux pattes sur le côté. Dos droit.

White tussor auto coat rimmed with half-belt on each side. Straight back.

Tailleur en lainage fantaisie garni de biais détachés, deux sur les côtés et un dans le dos.

Checked wool, trimmed with unfastened bias bands, two on side, one in back.

**SIMPLE BUT CHIC
THESE CREATIONS FROM
DOBB'S**

66, Avenue Victor-Hugo

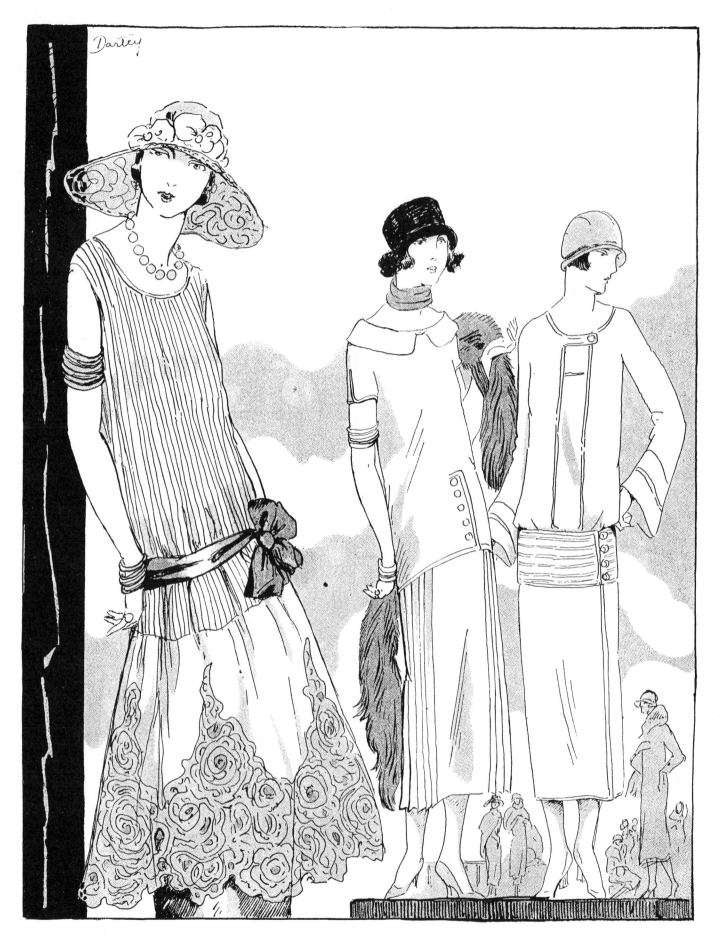

Robe plissée blanche, dentelle de soie rouge, dessous de Fulgurante rouge.

A white pleated gown, red silk lace, red Fulgurante slip.

MARTIAL ET ARMAND

Robe en jersey de soie blanche.

White silk jersey.

MOLYNEUX

Robe en Kasha blanc, soutaches de soie blanche.

White Kasha, white silk braid.

MOLYNEUX

FOR THE LAST FINE DAYS

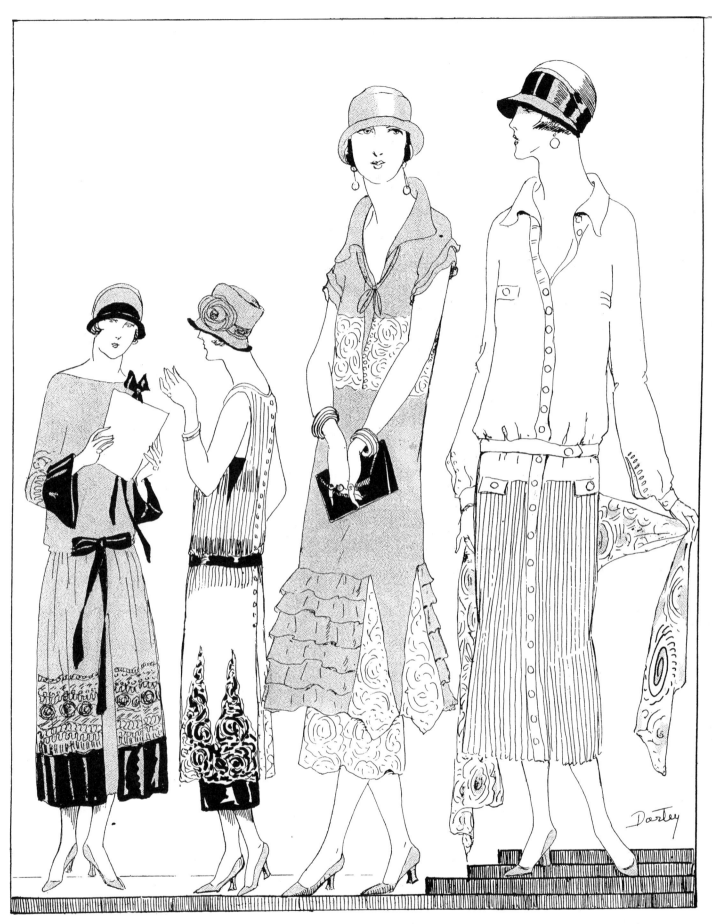

Robe en crêpe de Chine «rouille».
Satin noir, broderies blanches,
noires et «rouille».

Rust coloured crêpe de Chine.
Black satin, white, black and
rust coloured embroidery.

NICOLE GROULT

Robe en dentelle rouge
sur satin, le haut du
corsage en crêpe blanc.

Red lace over satin, the top of
the bodice made of white
crêpe.

MARTIAL ET ARMAND

Robe en crêpe
de Chine bleu,
et crêpe brodé.

Blue crêpe de
Chine, and em-
broidered crêpe

MADELEINE ET MADELEINE

Robe en crêpe
de Chine, uni
et plissé.

Plain and pleated
crêpe de Chine.

NICOLE GROULT

FOR THE LAST RAYS OF SUNLIGHT

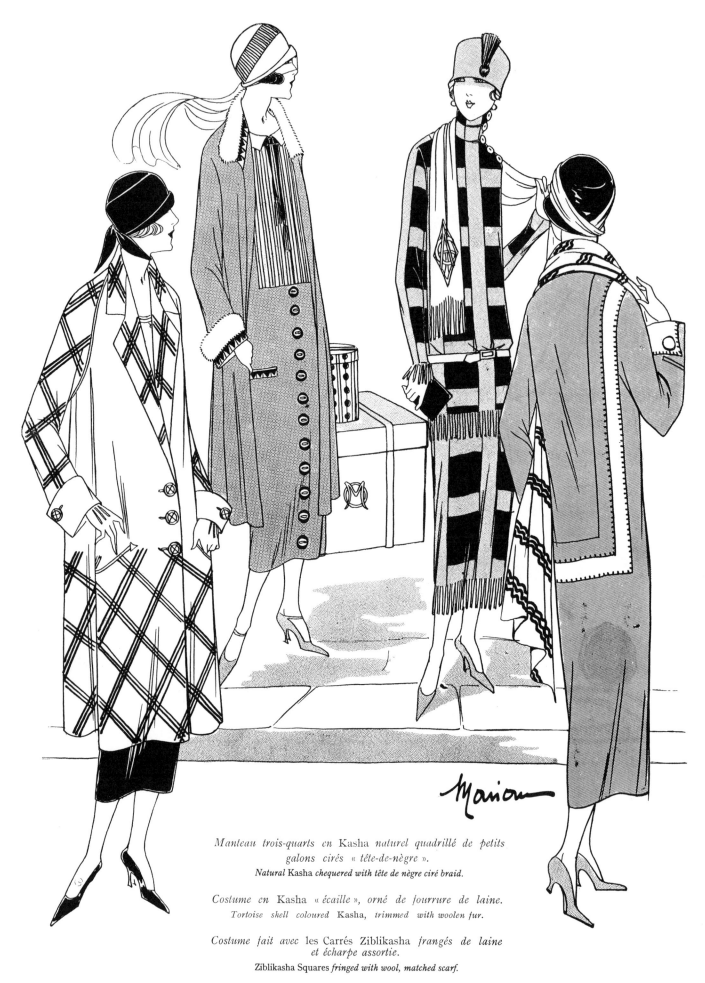

*Manteau trois-quarts en Kasha naturel quadrillé de petits
galons cirés « tête-de-nègre ».*
Natural Kasha chequered with tête de nègre ciré braid.

Costume en Kasha « écaille », orné de fourrure de laine.
Tortoise shell coloured Kasha, trimmed with woolen fur.

*Costume fait avec les Carrés Ziblikasha frangés de laine
et écharpe assortie.*
Ziblikasha Squares fringed with wool, matched scarf.

Manteau en Poplalga « sable », incrusté de même tissu rouge.
Sand coloured Poplalga, insets of same material in red.

AT THE DEPARTURE OF THE TRAIN BLEU
DEAUVILLE EXPRESS

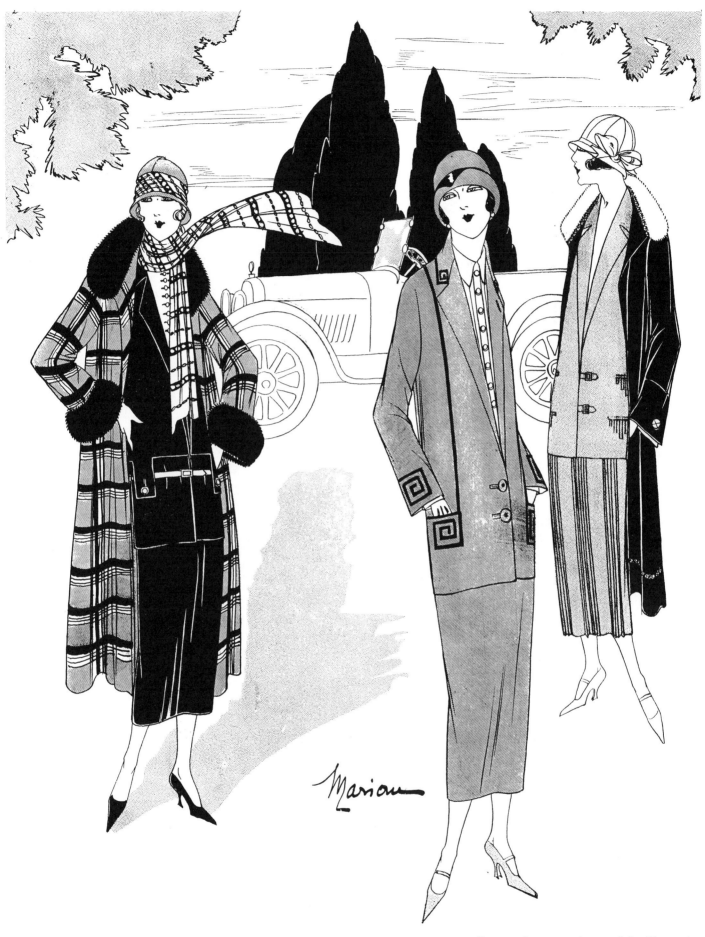

Costume en Kasha «*pain brûlé*», avec *liséré gris et petite ceinture de daim gris, manteau de Kasha écossais.*

Toast coloured Kasha, *with grey piping, grey suede belt. Plaid Kasha coat.*

Costume de Marokellaine *havane, garni de tresse cirée.*

Tobacco coloured Marokellaine, *trimmed with ciré braid.*

Costume de serge grise, *orné de plis, pattes et boucles. Manchette de Raillaine «brique» avec col en forme de laine assortie.*

Grey serge trimmed with pleats, straps and buckles. Brick *coloured Raillaine cuff with matched wool circular collar*

MERRY AUTOMOBILE JAUNTS

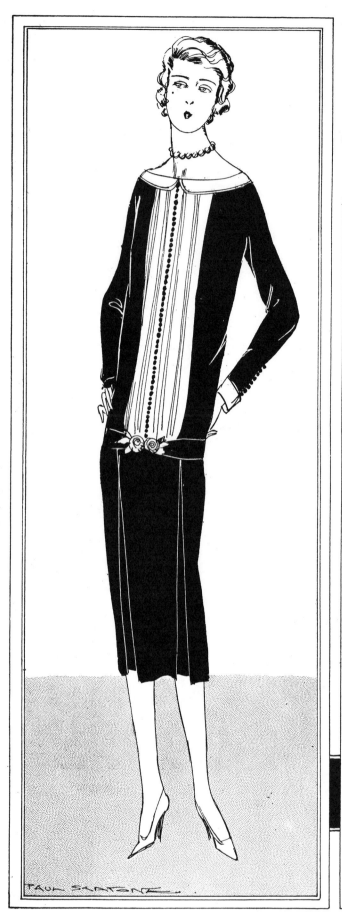

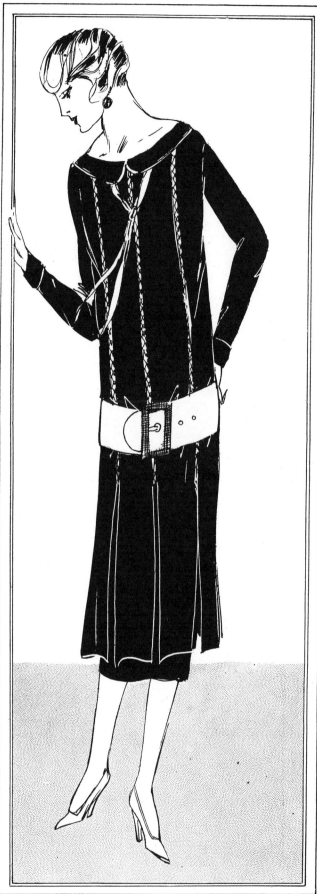

*Robe de Kasha « brique ». Gilet en crêpe
de Chine ocre plissé.*

Brick coloured Kasha, ochre coloured
pleated crêpe de Chine gilet.

*Robe de Marocain noir bordé vert éme-
raude, ceinture de peau de Suède noire.*

Black Marocain, edged with emerald
green, black suede belt.

TWO AFTERNOON DRESSES FROM
CARLY
7, Rue des Capucines

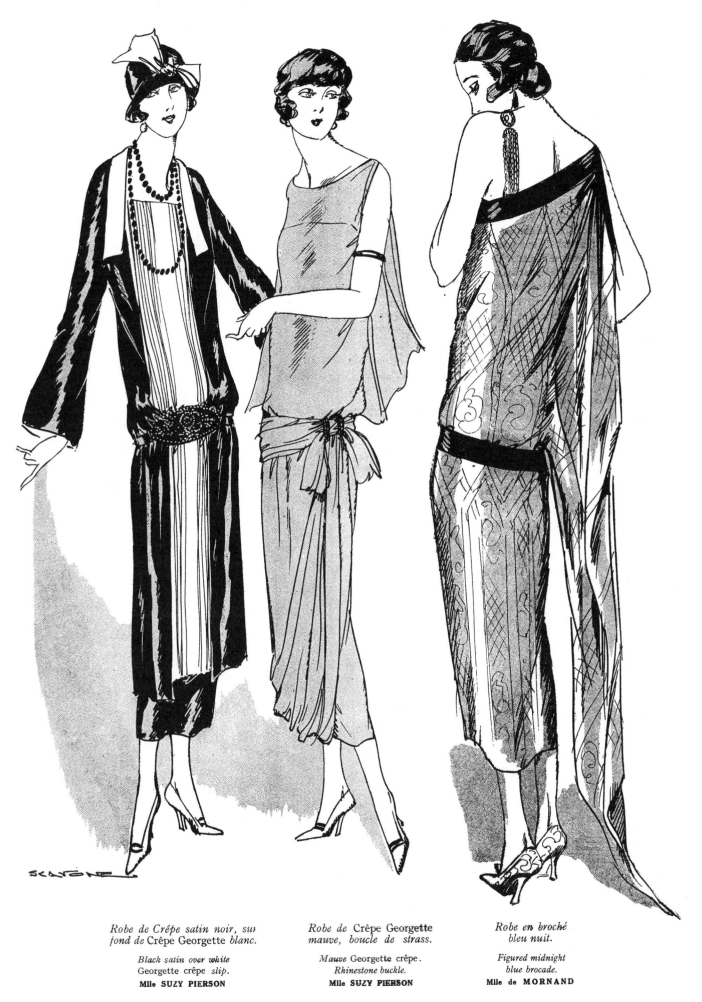

Robe de Crêpe satin noir, sur fond de Crêpe Georgette blanc.

Black satin over white
Georgette crêpe *slip.*
Mlle SUZY PIERSON

Robe de Crêpe Georgette mauve, boucle de strass.

Mauve Georgette crêpe.
Rhinestone buckle.
Mlle SUZY PIERSON

Robe en broché bleu nuit.

Figured midnight
blue brocade.
Mlle de MORNAND

AT *LE MARIAGE DE FREDAINE*, AT THE THÉÂTRE DE L'ÉTOILE, WE SKETCHED THESE

CREATIONS BY LUCIEN LELONG

16, Rue Matignon

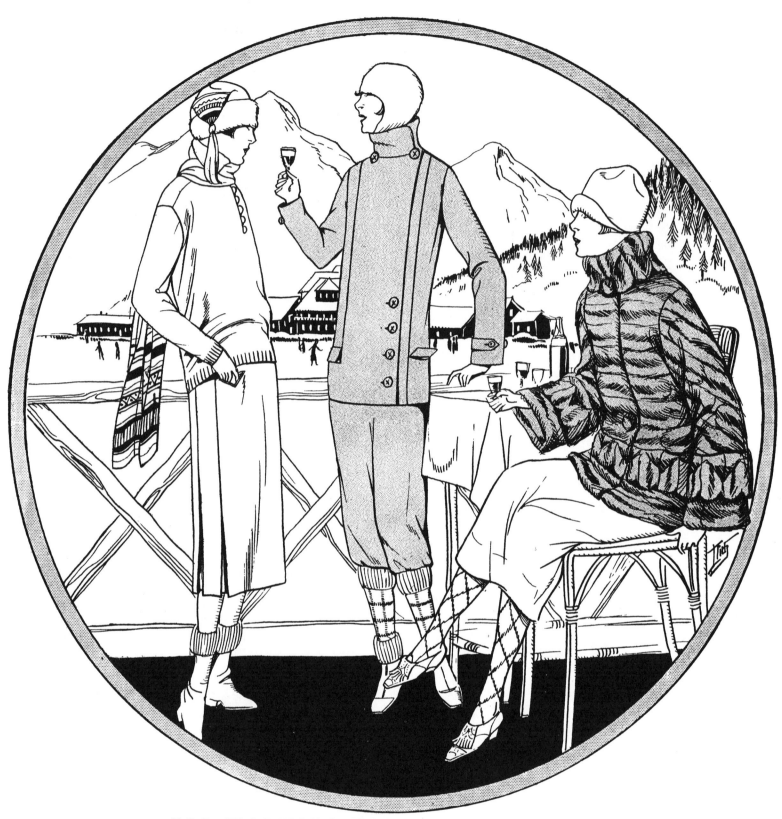

FOR WARMING YOURSELF A LITTLE

Jupe en Homespun vert vif, avec poches et double plis creux de chaque côté.

Bright green Homespun skirt with pockets, and two deep pleats on each side.

Veste de sport en Whipcord « fraise », col fermant hermétiquement, garnie de boutons de corozo, culotte assortie.

Strawberry coloured Whipcord sport jacket, funnel collar, trimmed with corozo buttons, matched trousers.

Petit paletot de taupe travaillé de façon nouvelle, avec bandes rapportées et dentelées ; bande du vêtement formant poches.

Mole fur worked in patterned bands, mole bands forming pockets.

WINTER SPORTS COSTUMES BY BUSVINE
48, Rue Pierre Charron

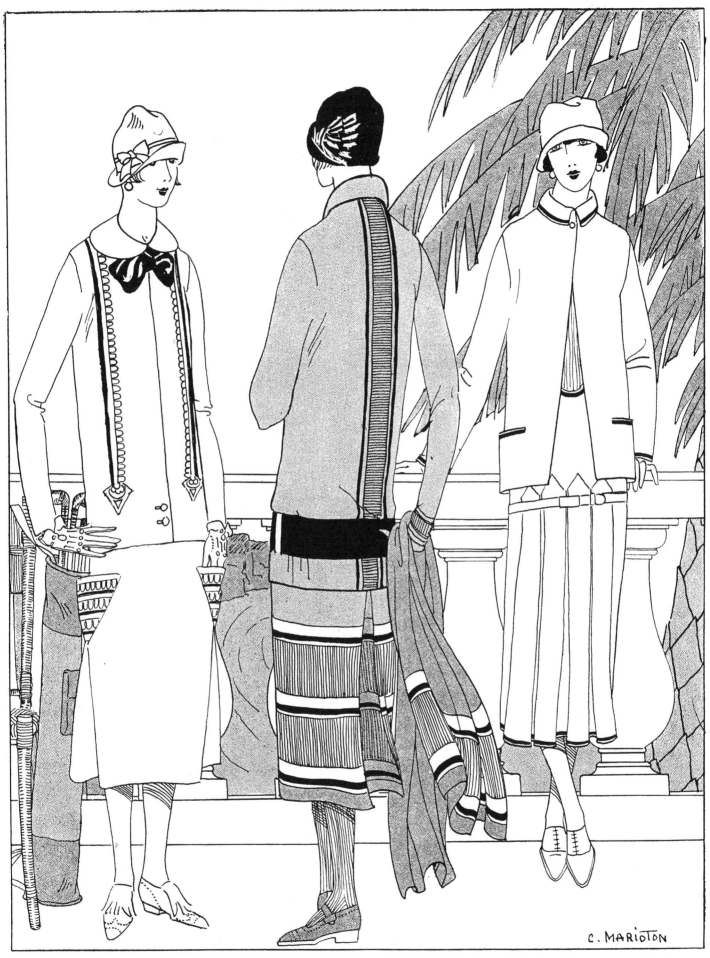

C. MARIOTON

Tailleur en drap blanc brodé vert et rouge ; cravate verte ; jupe en forme.

White wool, embroidered in green and red, green cravat, circular skirt.

Tailleur en Kasha beige, garni 'de\bandes en même tissu bleu, noir et blanc. Large ceinture en daim bleu.

Beige Kasha, *trimmed with blue, black and white Kasha bands, wide blue suede belt.*

Robe trois pièces en serge blanche bordée d'un biais blanc et rouge. Gilet d'Organdina plissé.

Serge, white and red piping, pleated Organdina gilet.

LE SPORT ON THE CÔTE D'AZUR

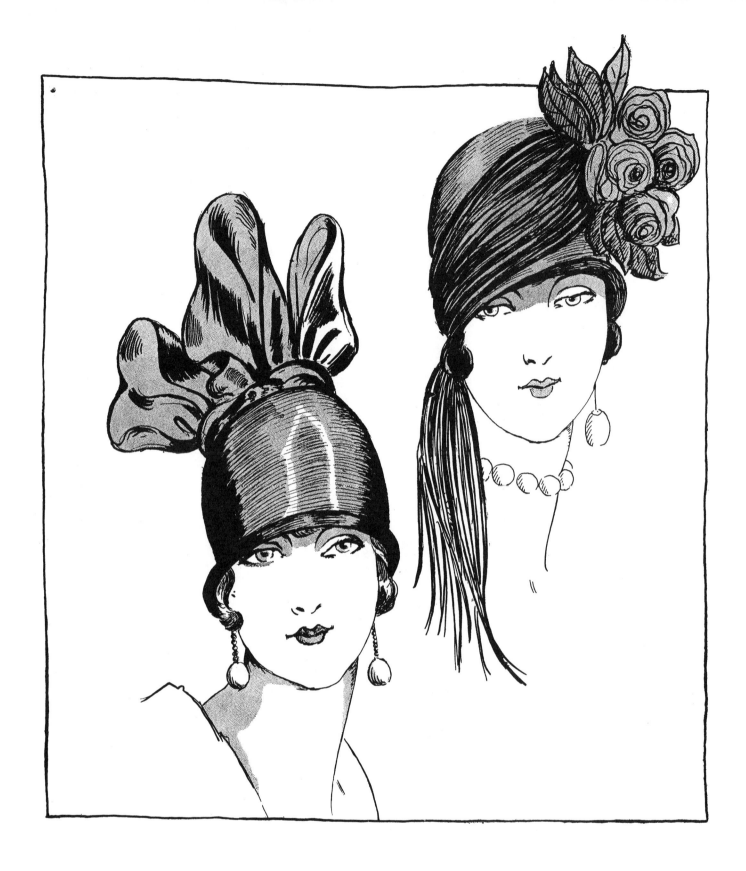

*Chapeau en picot **vert**
et ruban du même ton.*

*Green picot straw **and**
matching ribbon hat.*

*Crin «vert amande» foncé,
roses rouges, feuillage vert.*

*Dark almond green horsehair
hat, red roses, green leaves.*

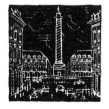 C H E Z   M A R I A   G U Y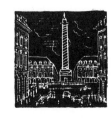

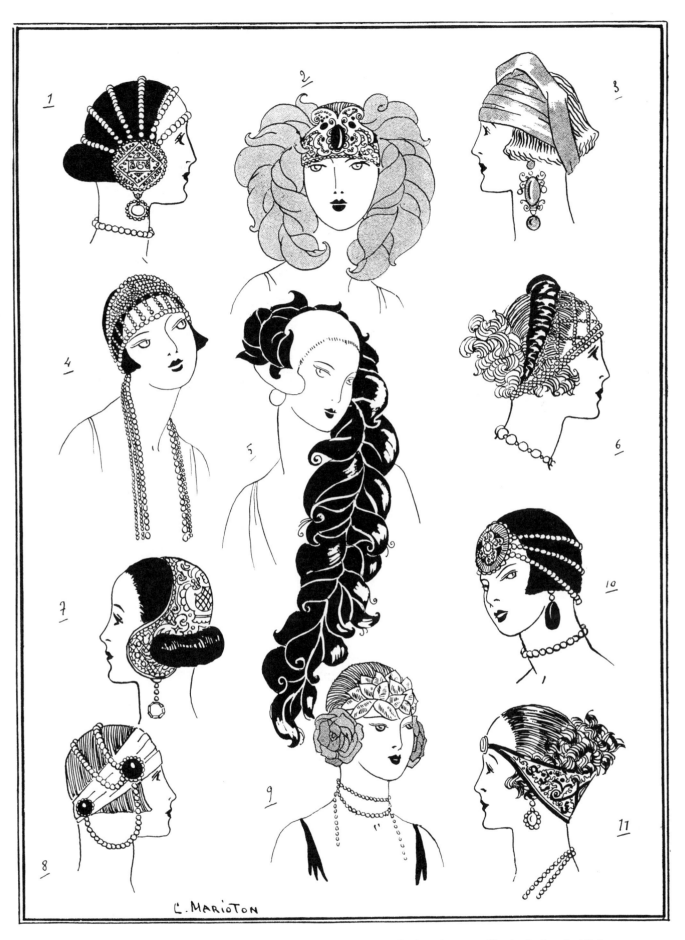

L. MARIOTON

1. Strands of pearls held on the ears by roundels embroidered with pearls and rhinestones, ending in earrings.   2. Silver lamé and amethyst diadem; mauve ostrich plumes.   3. Green and gold lamé turban, long matching earrings.   4. Iridescent pearl diadem.   5. Long ostrich plume passing behind the head and falling over one shoulder.   6. Lattice of pearls, padded band of silver lamé.   7. Small cap of gold tulle, bead and gold embroidery.   8. White velvet bandeau; beads and blue cabochons.   9. Silver leaves and red and pink velvet roses.   10. Black and white enamel roundel securing three strands of pearls.   11. Black and white pearls embroidered on nasturtium velvet.

IDEA OF THE WEEK: EVENING HEADDRESSES

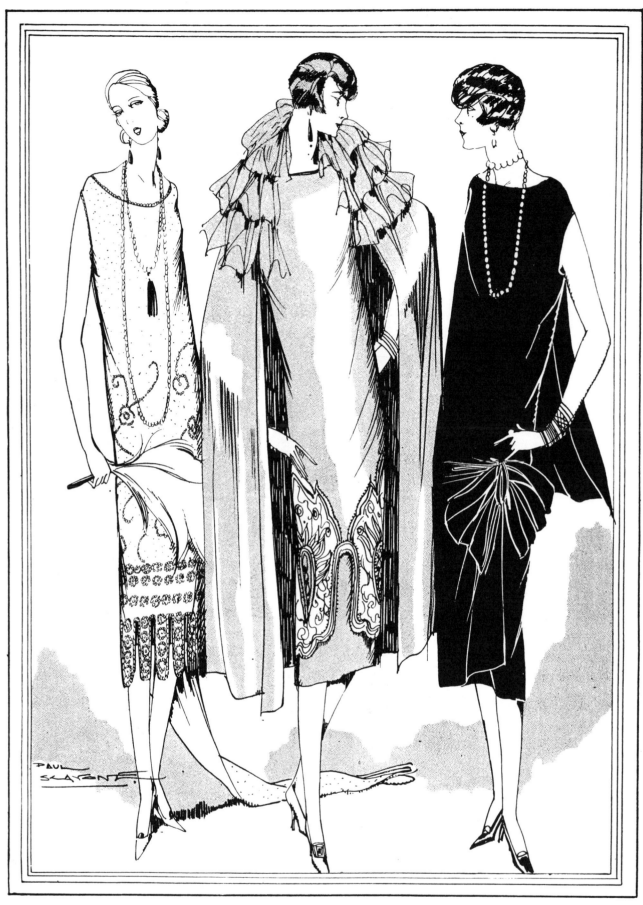

Robe du soir, en crêpe
satin blanc, brodée de
tubes d'or et diamants.

Dress of white satin crêpe
embroidered with gold bugle
beads and brilliants.

Ensemble du soir en panne Sésostris
« rose buvard », perles et cabochons
en nacre de ton lavande.

Evening ensemble of blotting-paper pink
Sèsostris velvet, lavender mother of pearl
beads and ornaments.

Robe de panne noire,
garnie d'un gros nœud
formant drapé.

Black velvet gown,
trimmed with large
bow forming drape.

AT A GALA DINNER AT THE AMBASSADEURS
IN CANNES
CREATIONS FROM MOLYNEUX

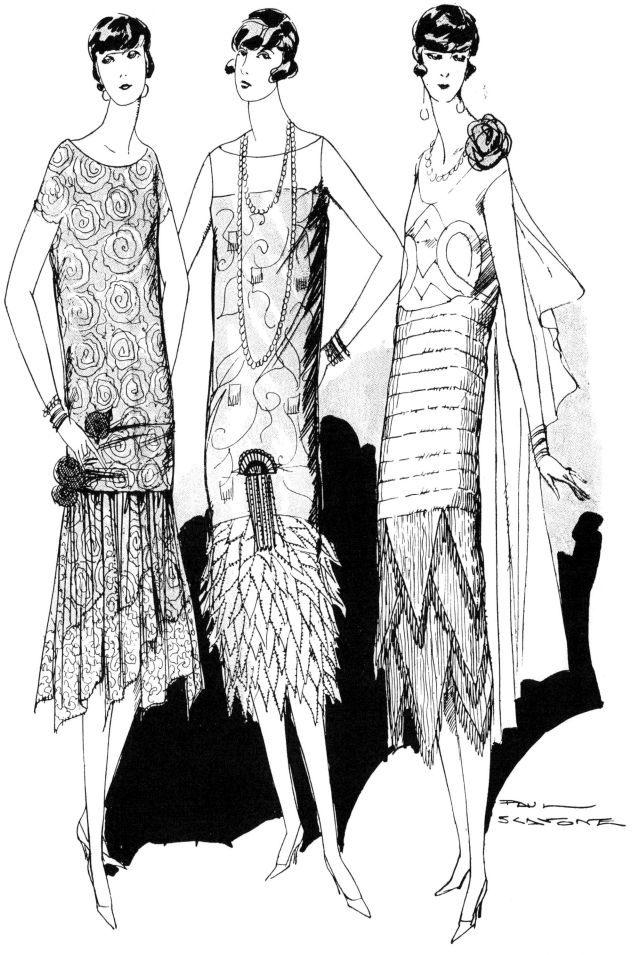

Robe de dentelle beige
sur fond ivoire.

Beige lace gown over
ivory slip.

Robe de dentelle d'or sur fond de
Fulgurante *rose et pointes brodées.*

Gold lace gown over pink Fulgurante
slip, and embroidered points.

Robe de tulle, brodée de
tubes et strass

Tulle gown embroidered with
bugle beads and rhinestones.

Mlle. DARTY, IN UNE FEMME [A WOMAN] AT THE THÉÂTRE FEMINA,

WEARS THESE OUTFITS BY CALLOT

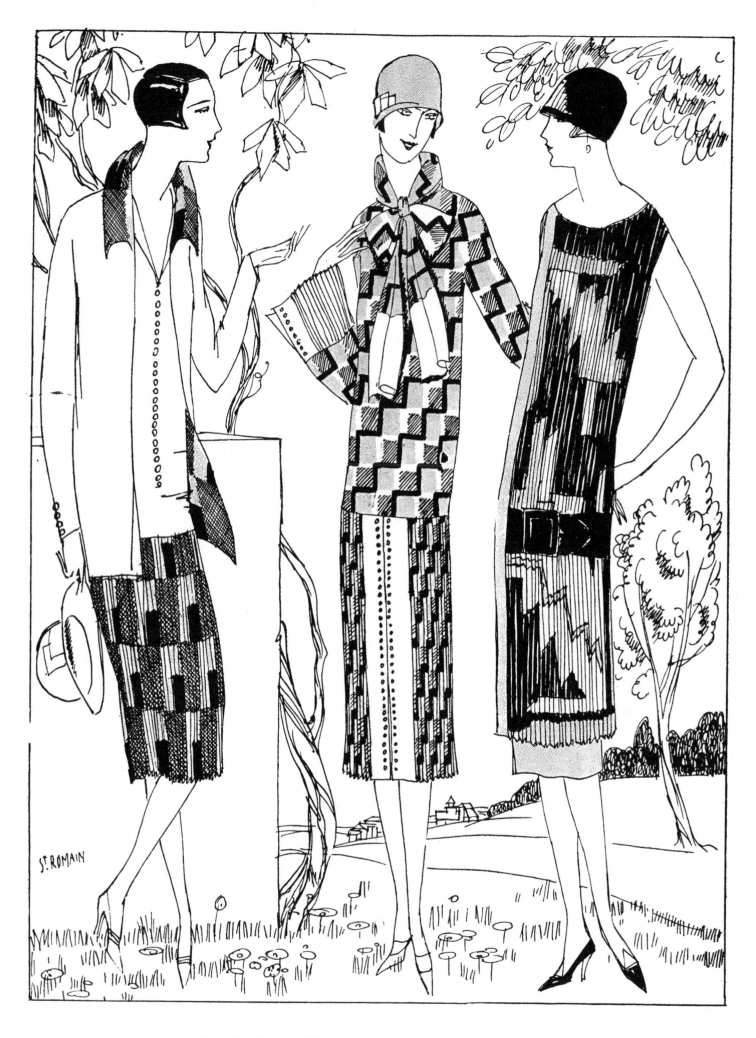

CUBISM HAS INSPIRED THESE NEW FABRICS
CREATIONS BY GODAU, GUILLAUME

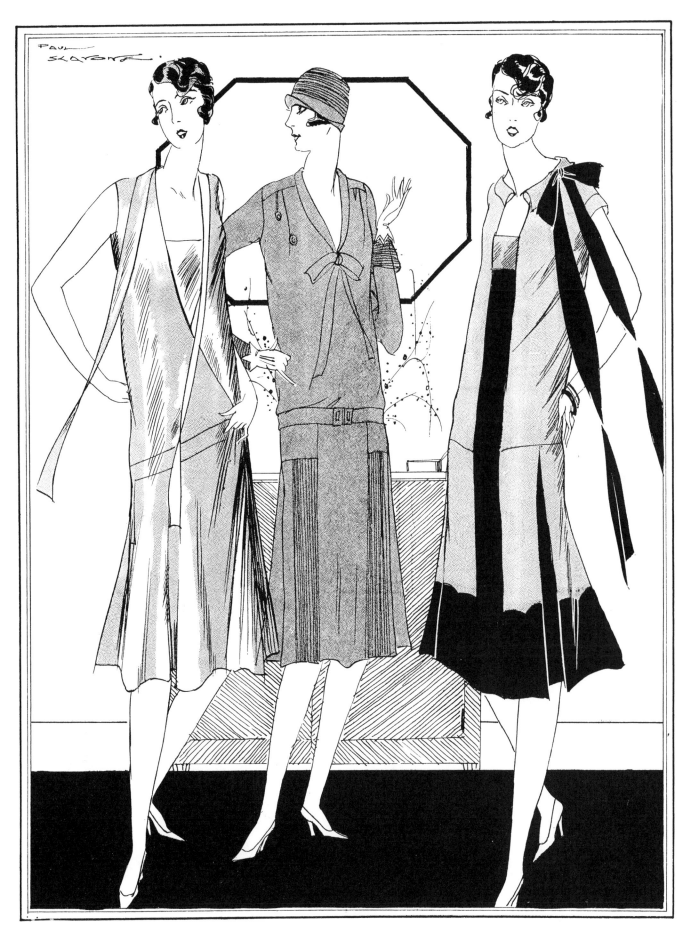

Robe de crêpe satin mauve rose.

Pink mauve satin crêpe gown.

Robe de reps de soie « bois de rose ».

« Bois de rose » coloured silk rep gown.

Robe de crêpe de Chine et Georgette « amande » de deux tons.

Two shades of almond coloured crêpe de Chine and Georgette gown.

THE OUTFITS OF Mlle. S. DULAC IN *LE MARIAGE DE MAMAN* [MAMA'S WEDDING] AT THE THÉÂTRE ANTOINE

CREATIONS BY JEAN PATOU

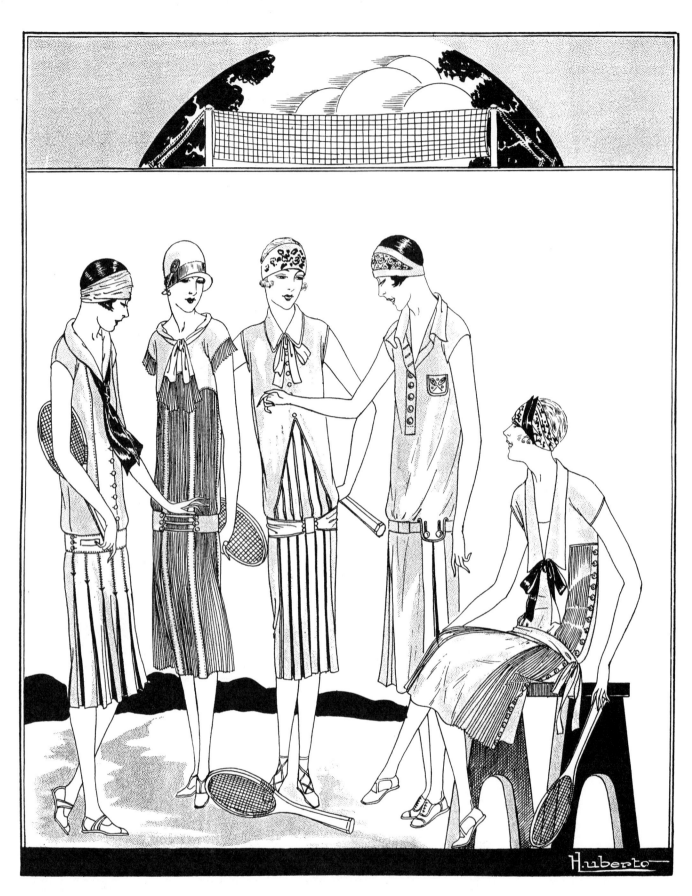

Robe en Kasha blanc, col et devant de piqué blanc, boutons de nacre, cravate marine.

White Kasha dress, white piqué front and collar, mother-of-pearl buttons, navy blue tie.

Robe en crêpe Tantale blanc finement plissé, encolure nouée terminée par du plissé.

White Tantale crêpe dress, finely pleated, knotted neck-opening ending in pleats.

Robe en crêpe Athénien blanc, incrustation de plis ronds sur le devant seulement, col rabattu, cravate nouée, boucle d'argent.

White Crepella dress, buttonhole placket, leather belt, two pleats on each side.

Robe en Crépella blanc, patte-boutonnière, ceinture de peau, deux plis ronds de chaque côté.

White Crepella dress, buttonhole placket, leather belt, two pleats on each side.

Robe en piqué de soie blanc finement plissée sur les côtés, cravate en ruban de couleur boutons de nacre.

White silk piqué gown finely pleated on the side, coloured ribbon tie, mother-of-pearl buttons.

TENNIS REMAINS THE FAVOURITE SPORT OF WOMEN

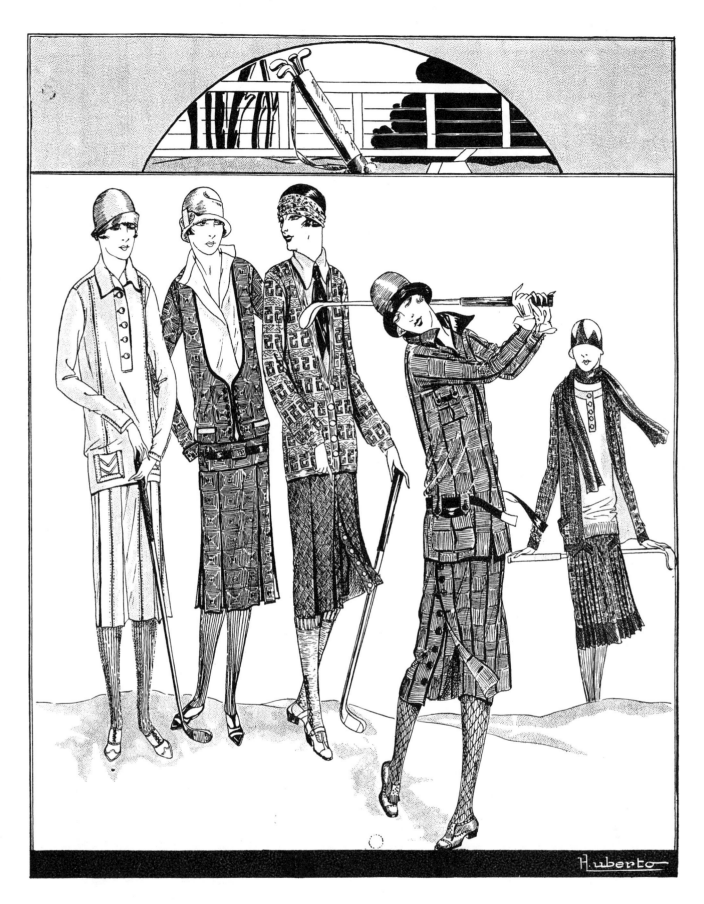

Ensemble composé d'un sweater et d'une jupe en Kasha beige.

Beige Kasha skirt and sweater.

Robe en Les Dalles losanges Filetta bordé de cuir, ceinture et boutons. Gilet de piqué blanc.

Les Dalles Filletta dress, leather edging, belt and buttons, white piqué gilet.

Sweater de laine brodé de couleurs vives, jupe de lainage sur culotte en taffetas bois de rose, chemisier de linon, cravate de faille.

Wool sweater embroidered in bright colours, woolen material skirt over «bois de rose» taffeta culottes, lawn blouse, faille tie.

Tailleur en Rayures Filetta, poches à soufflet, garnies de peau, culotte indépendante.

Striped Filletta suit, pockets trimmed with leather, separate culottes.

Ensemble en Damiers Natella beige moucheté, chandail en laine blanche, écharpe, bas de jupe et bordure en tissu rouge.

Beige spotted Damiers Natella ensemble, white wool sweater, scarf, hem and borders in red.

ON THE LINKS' GREEN CARPET

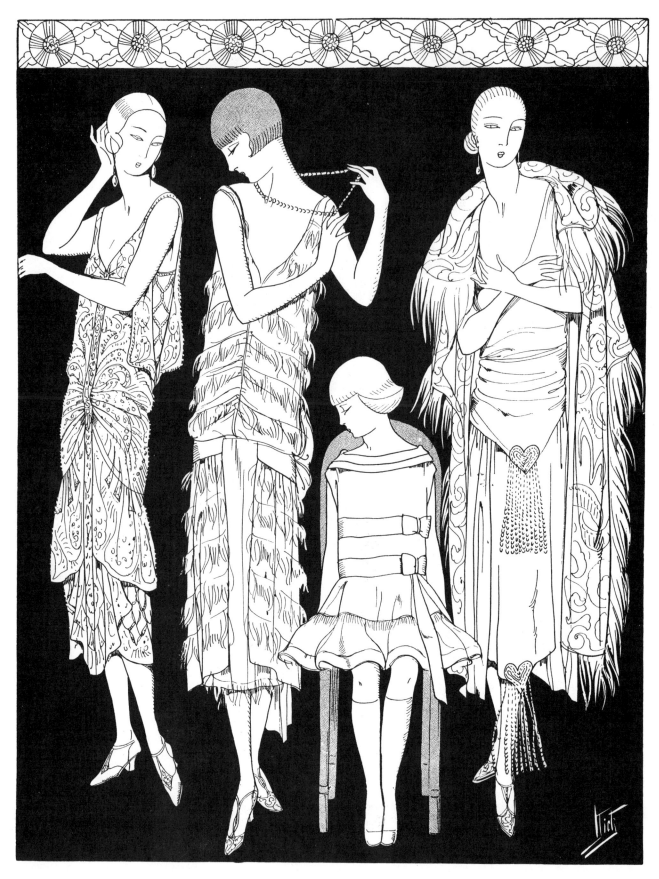

Robe en crêpe blanc, perlée de brillants et cristal ; mouvement drapé devant.

White crêpe gown, beaded with diamonds and crystal, draped in the front.

Robe de crêpe blanc, garnie de petites franges en filigranne d'argent, mouvement de tunique ouverte devant.

White Georgette gown, trimmed with fine silver fringes, tunic opened at the front.

Robe de fillette, en crêpe blanc, garnie de larges rubans de satin, avec nœuds sur le côté.

Young girl's gown of white crêpe, trimmed with wide satin ribbon and bows on side.

Robe de satin blanc, garnie de motifs et chutes de perles, cape en lamé blanc et argent frangée de singe blanc.

White satin gown, trimmed with ornaments and fringe of pearls, white and silver lamé cape, edged with white monkey.

AT "LA COLLECTIVITÉ DE LA COUTURE"
MODELS FROM PAQUIN

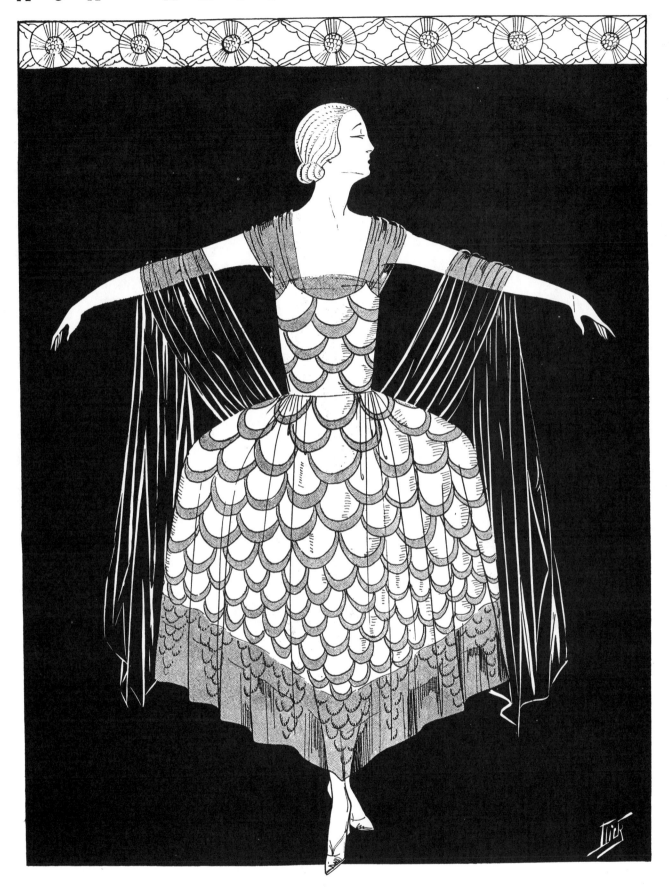

*Robe de style, faite d'écailles
d'argent sur tulle noir,
grande écharpe de tulle noir.*

*Robe de style, silver scales over
black tulle, long black tulle scarf.*

AT THE "COLLECTIVITÉ DE LA COUTURE"
MODEL FROM MADELEINE VIONNET

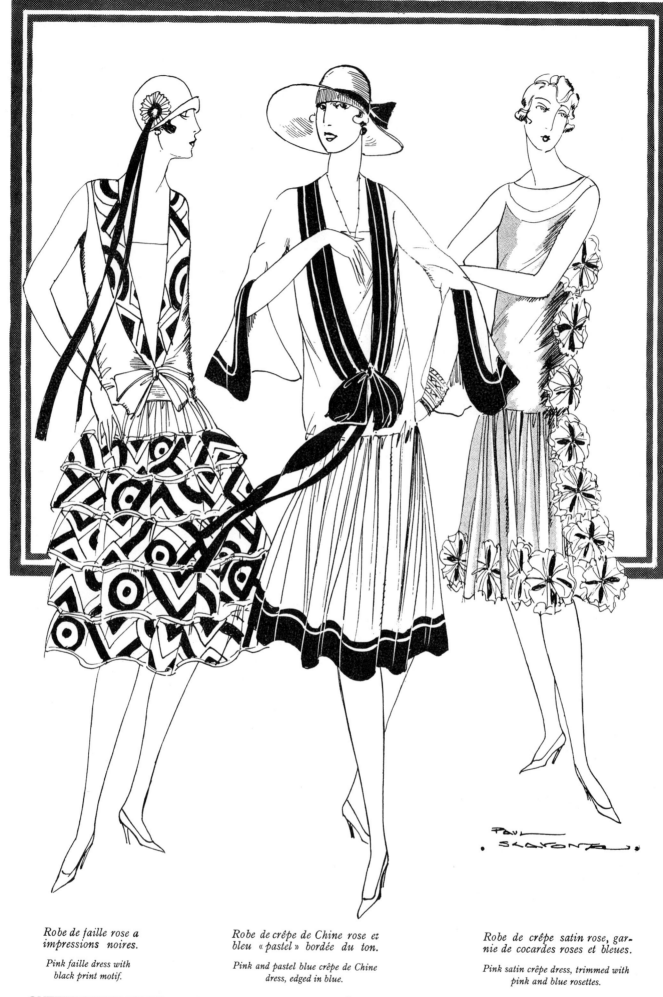

*Robe de faille rose a
impressions noires.*

Pink faille dress with
black print motif.

*Robe de crêpe de Chine rose et
bleu «pastel» bordée du ton.*

Pink and pastel blue crêpe de Chine
dress, edged in blue.

*Robe de crêpe satin rose, gar-
nie de cocardes roses et bleues.*

Pink satin crêpe dress, trimmed with
pink and blue rosettes.

OUTFITS WORN BY Mlle. MAGUY VARNA IN *BOUCHE À BOUCHE* [MOUTH TO MOUTH] **AT THE APOLLO**
CREATIONS BY JEANNE LANVIN

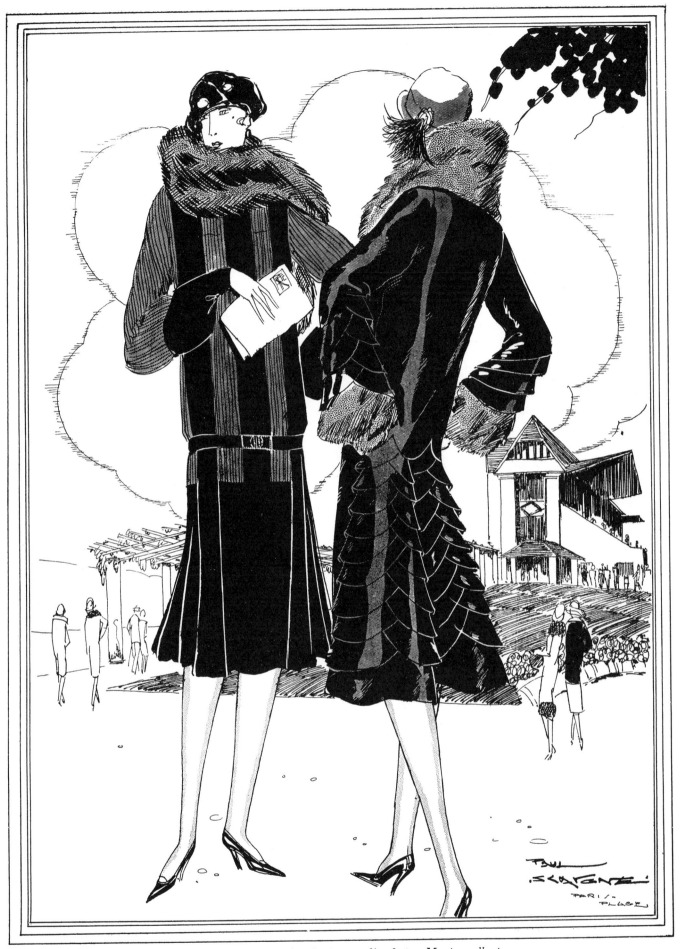

Robe de velours de soie noir et mousseline du ton. Manteau allant
avec la robe en Fulgurante noire, bas de manches et col de zibeline.

Black silk velvet and chiffon dress. Matching coat of black
Fulgurante with sable collar and cuffs.

SEEN AT THE RACES AT LE TOUQUET, TWO DRESSES BY
C Y B E R
4, Place de l'Opéra

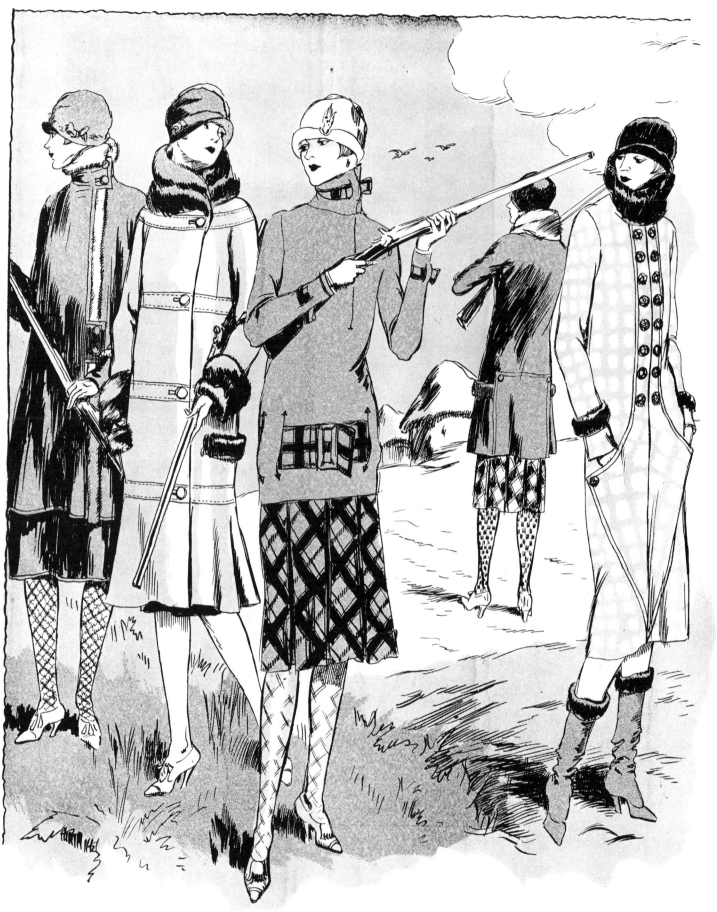

Costume en cuir bleu, doublé de fourrure.

Blue leather costume, lined with fur.

Manteau en velours beige, doublé et orné de loutre.

Beige velvet coat, lined and trimmed with otter.

Jupe en tartan écossais, corsage en velours du ton.

Plaid tartan skirt, matching velvet blouse.

Veste en cuir noir et fourrure grise. Jupe écossaise.

Black leather jacket, grey fur. Plaid skirt.

Manteau en tartan rouille et gris, orné de fourrure.

Rust coloured and grey tartan coat, trimmed with fur.

A DAY'S HUNTING IN SCOTLAND
OUTFITS FOR DAY AND EVENING

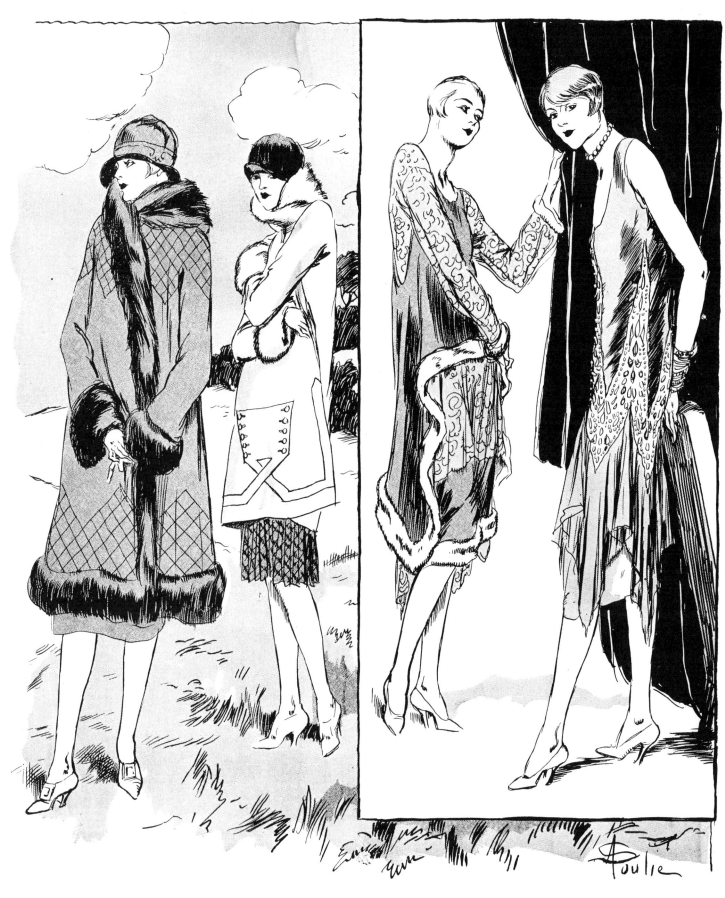

Manteau ample en velours corduroy bleu, orné de piqûres et de fourrure.

Full blue corduroy coat, trimmed with stitching and fur.

Manteau en tartan beige avec poche devant.

Beige tartan coat with pocket in front.

Après la chasse : déshabillé en velours et dentelle.

After the hunt : velvet and lace « déshabillé ».

Robe du soir en lamé argent, recouverte de mousseline bleu paon, avec applications de pierreries.

Silver lamé evening gown, covered with peacock blue chiffon, appliquéd jewels.

CREATIONS BY REVILLE

(DRESSMAKER TO HER MAJESTY QUEEN MARY OF ENGLAND)

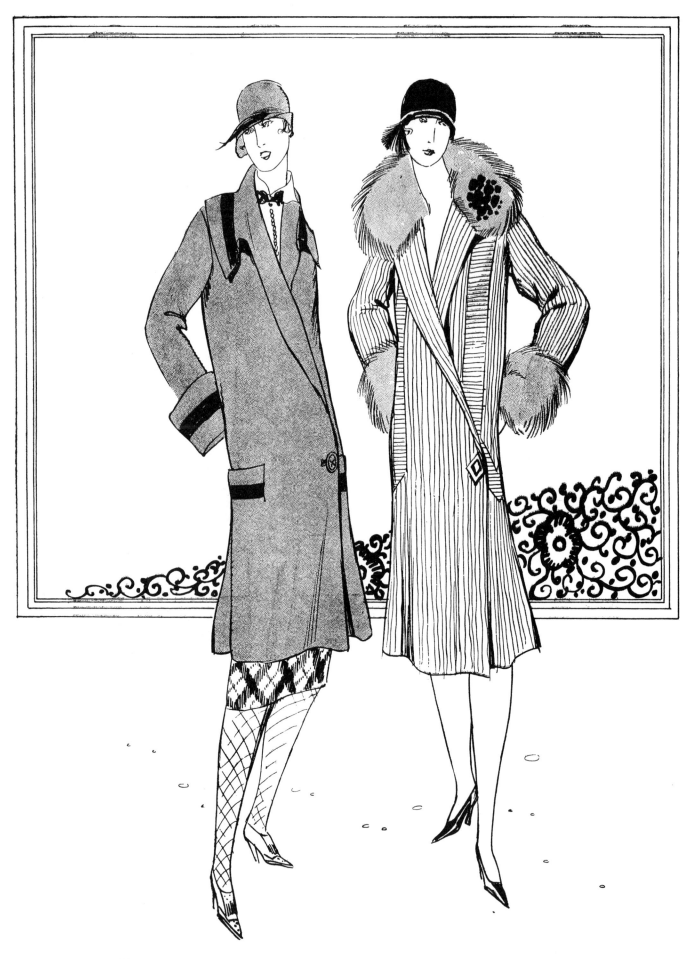

*Manteau de lainage «réséda» et incrustations
de peau verte.*

Reseda coloured wool coat, with green leather insets.

*Manteau de velours de laine côtelé
beige, fourrure du ton.*

Beige ribbed woolen velvet, matching fur.

CHEZ CARLY

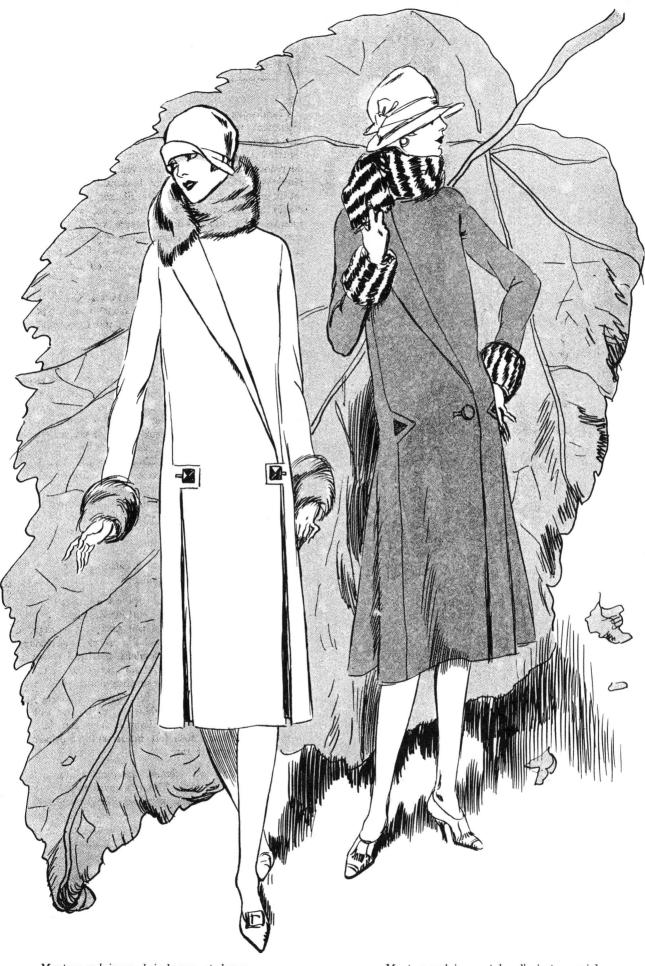

Manteau en lainage « bois de rose » et skungs décoloré.

«Bois de rose» coloured woolen coat trimmed
with bleached skunk.

Manteau en lainage « tabac d'orient » garni de zorinos noir à raies blanches.

Tobacco coloured woolen coat trimmed with
black sorinos with white stripes.

FOR AUTUMN, TWO OVERCOATS FROM DOBB'S

66, Avenue Victor-Hugo

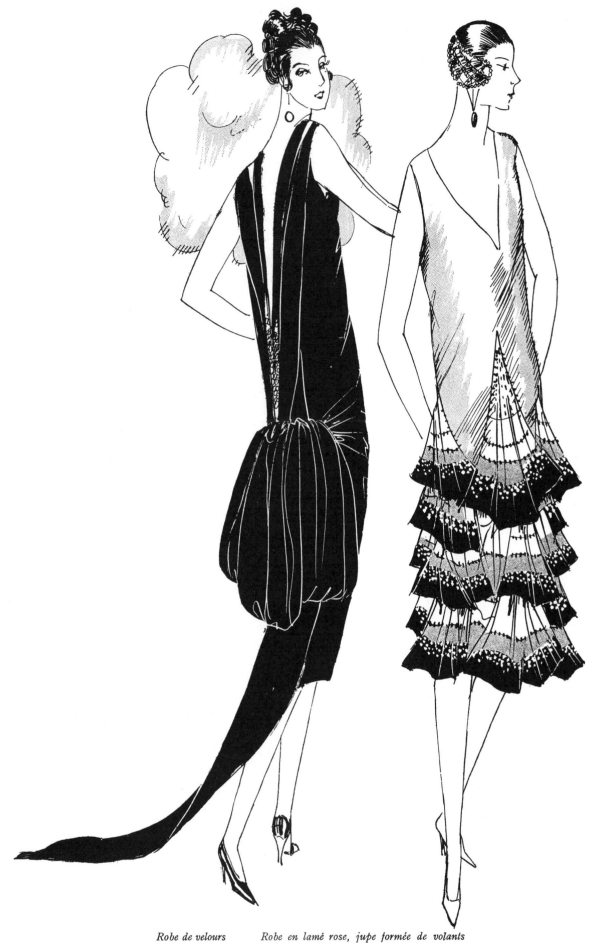

Robe de velours
vert d'eau.

Robe en lamé rose, jupe formée de volants
irréguliers en lamé rouge et or brodés de strass.

Sea green velvet
gown.

Pink lamé gown, skirt made of irregular flounces in red
and gold lamé, embroidered with rhinestones.

MADEMOISELLE SPINELLY, IN *UN DÉJEUNER DE SOLEIL* [LUNCHEON IN THE SUN]
AT THE COMÉDIE CAUMARTIN, WEARS THESE TWO GOWNS BY
L O U I S E B O U L A N G E R
3, Rue de Berri.

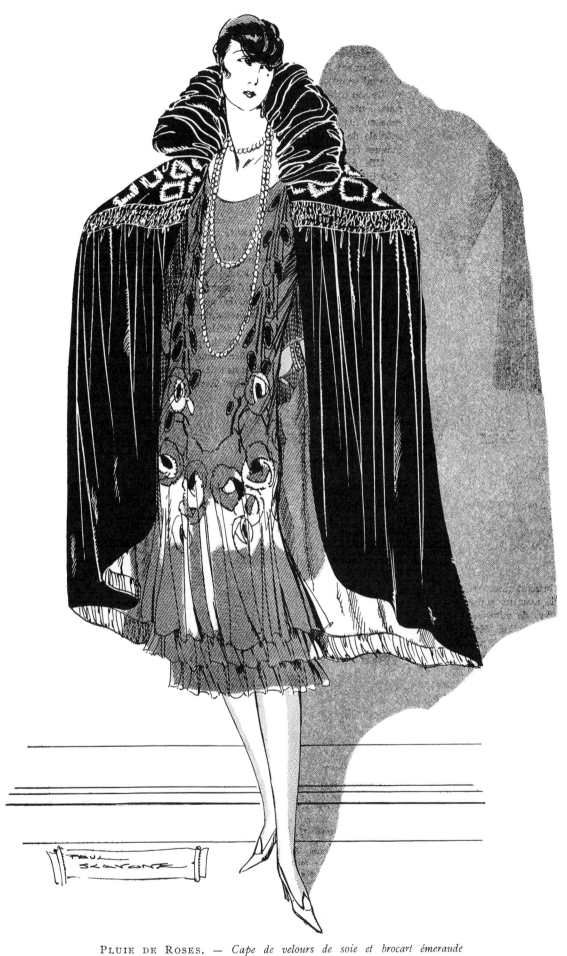

PLUIE DE ROSES. — *Cape de velours de soie et brocart émeraude sur une robe de mousseline imprimée, le haut vert et le bas rose dégradé.*

RAIN OF ROSES.—Emerald silk velvet and brocade cape, over a printed chiffon dress, the upper part green and the lower part in shades of pink.

FOR EVENING, THIS CREATION FROM CYBER
4, Place de l'Opéra, 4.

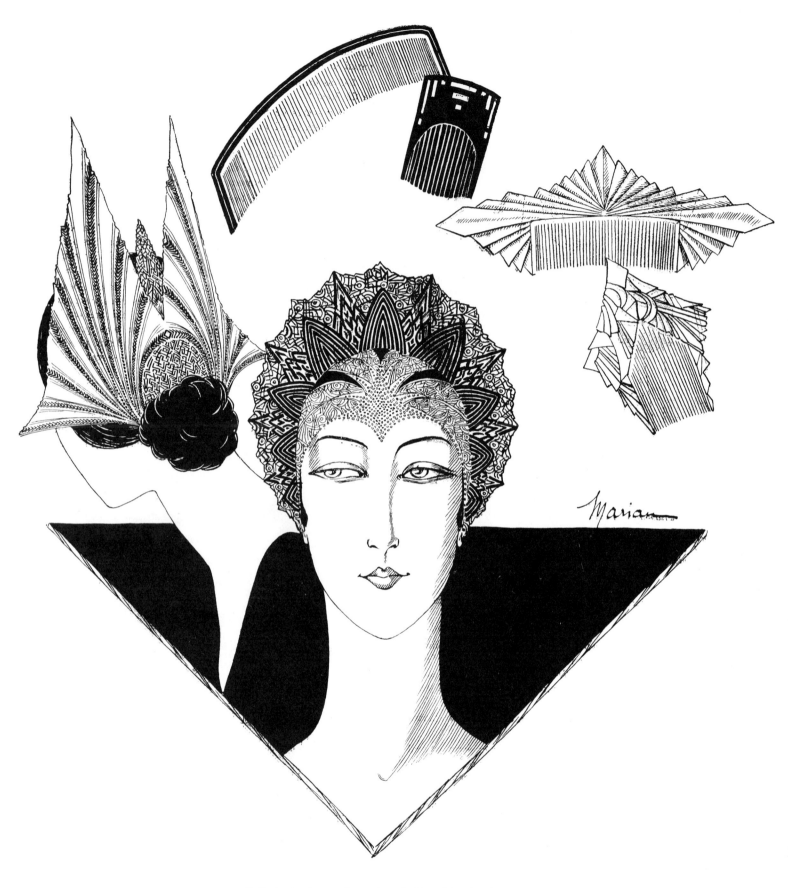

At the party given on June 16 at the Exposition des Arts Décoratifs, the combs in the "Caprice Espagnol" number, all suppled by Auguste Bonaz, were much admired. These combs can also be seen at the Grand Palais, divisions 9 and 20.

THE COMBS OF AUGUSTE BONAZ

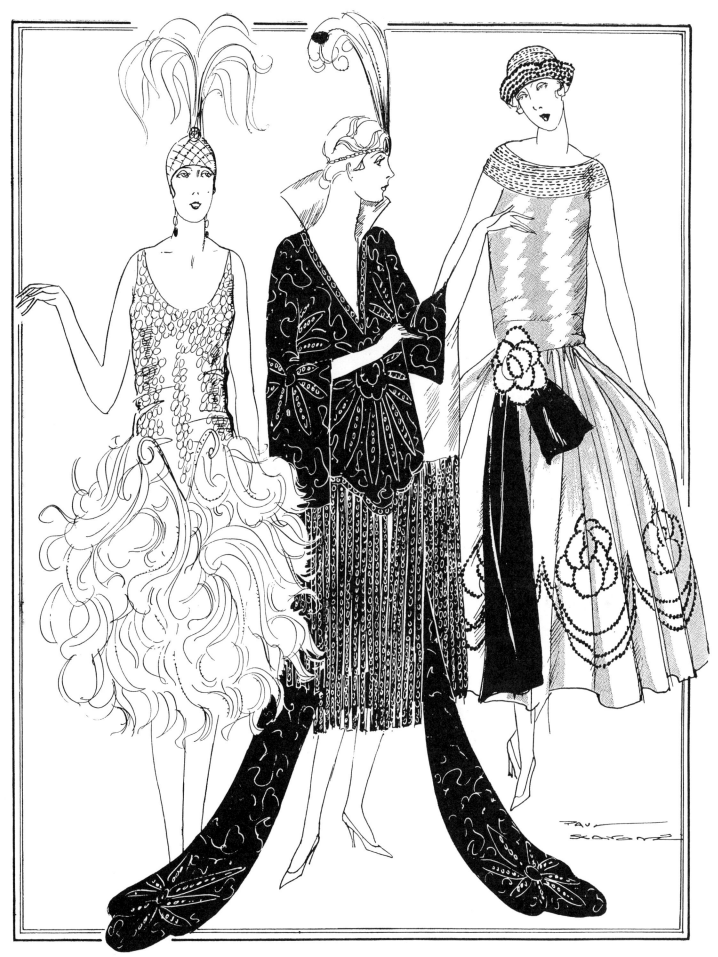

Robe-corselet en lamé
« cuivre » et paradis.

Copper coloured lamé gown
with bird of paradise plumes.

Robe de Marocain vert, doublée de lamé
d'argent, brodée d'argent et de sequins.

Green Marocain gown, lined with silver
lamé, embroidered with silver and sequins.

Robe de satin « corail » et nœud bleu
ciel, broderie de perles de corail.

Coral coloured satin gown, with sky
blue bow, coral bead embroidery.

THE OUTFITS OF Mlle. LUCIENNE DE LAHAYE IN *LA REVUE MISTINGUETT* AT THE MOULIN ROUGE

CREATIONS BY JEANNE LANVIN

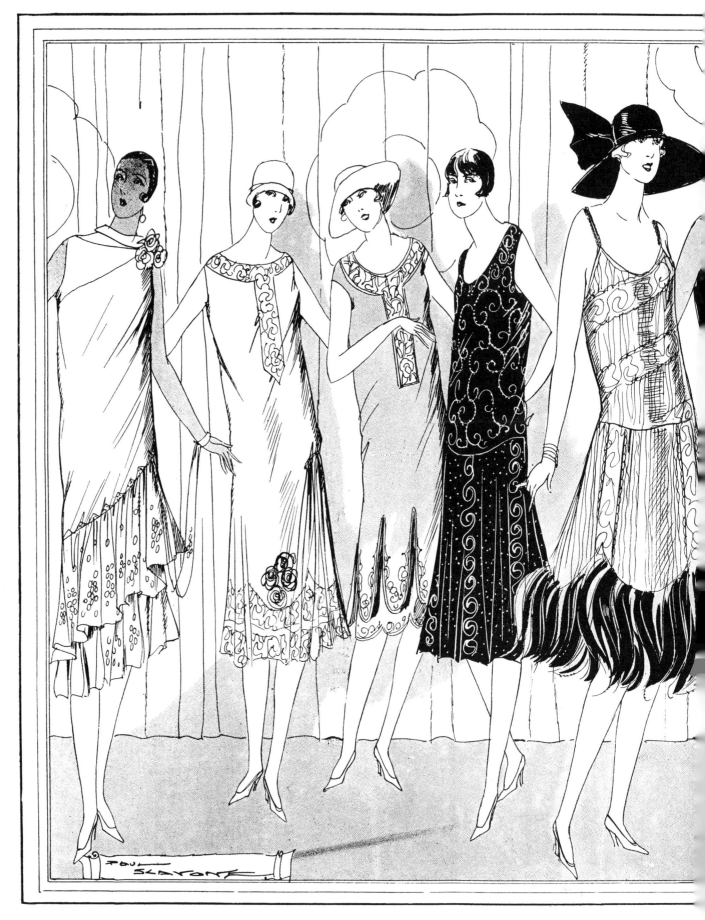

Robe de satin blanc, brodée d'argent.	Robe en crêpe «bois de rose» garnie de dentelle du ton.	Robe en crêpe rose et peau d'or.	Robe en velours de soie rose, brodée de strass.	Robe de lamé d'argent brodée de strass, bas de plume d'autruche verte.
White satin gown embroidered in silver.	*« Bois de rose » coloured crêpe gown, trimmed with matching lace.*	*Pink crêpe and gold leather gown.*	*Pink silk velvet gown, embroidered with rhinestones.*	*Silver lamé gown, embroidered with rhinestones, trimmed with green ostrich plumes.*
BEER	**MARTIAL ET ARMAND**	**MARTIAL et ARMAND**	**JEAN PATOU**	**MARTIAL ET ARMAND**

THE OUTFITS WORN IN *PARIS EN FLEURS* [PARIS

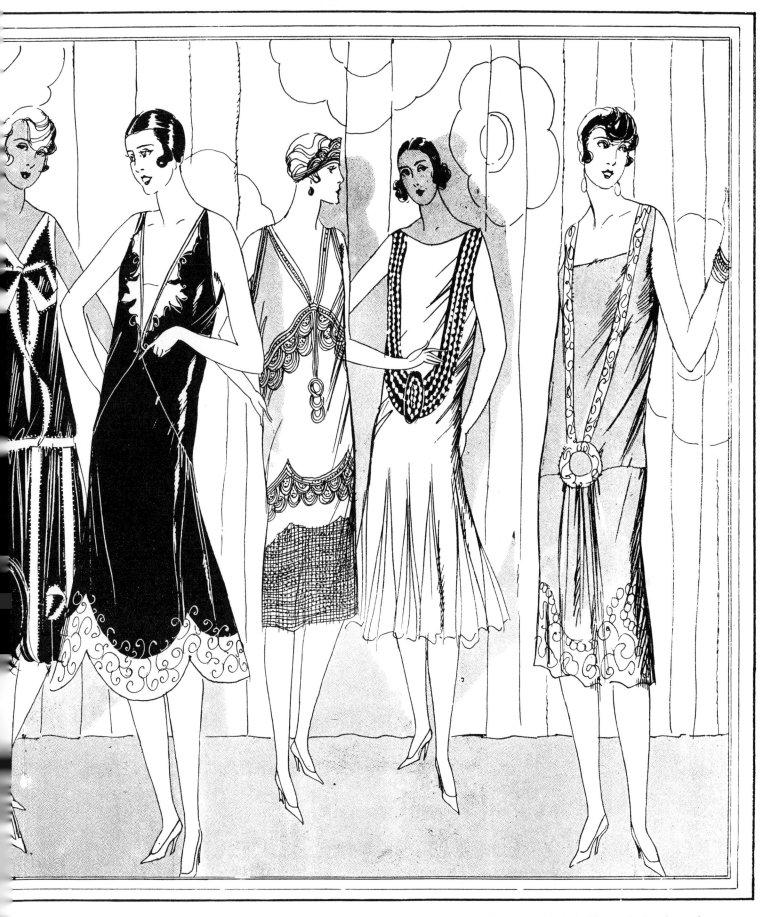

Robe de mousseline bleu sur
un fond de lamé d'argent.

*Blue chiffon gown
over silver lamé slip.*

MARTIAL ET ARMAND

Robe de velours de soie noir,
broderie de fleurs bleu et argent.

*Black silk velvet gown, blue
and silver flower embroidery.*

PREMET

Robe grise en crêpe satin,
broderie blanche et bleue.

*Grey satin crêpe gown,
white and blue embroidery.*

LUCIEN LELONG

Robe de Georgette violacé, brodée
de perles blanches sur fond bleu.

*Purple Georgette gown, embroidered
with white beads over blue slip.*

JEANNE LANVIN

Robe de velours vieux rose,
brodée de perles et de strass.

*Antique pink velvet gown, embroi-
dered with beads and rhinestones.*

JEAN PATOU

ECKED IN FLOWERS] AT THE CASINO DE PARIS

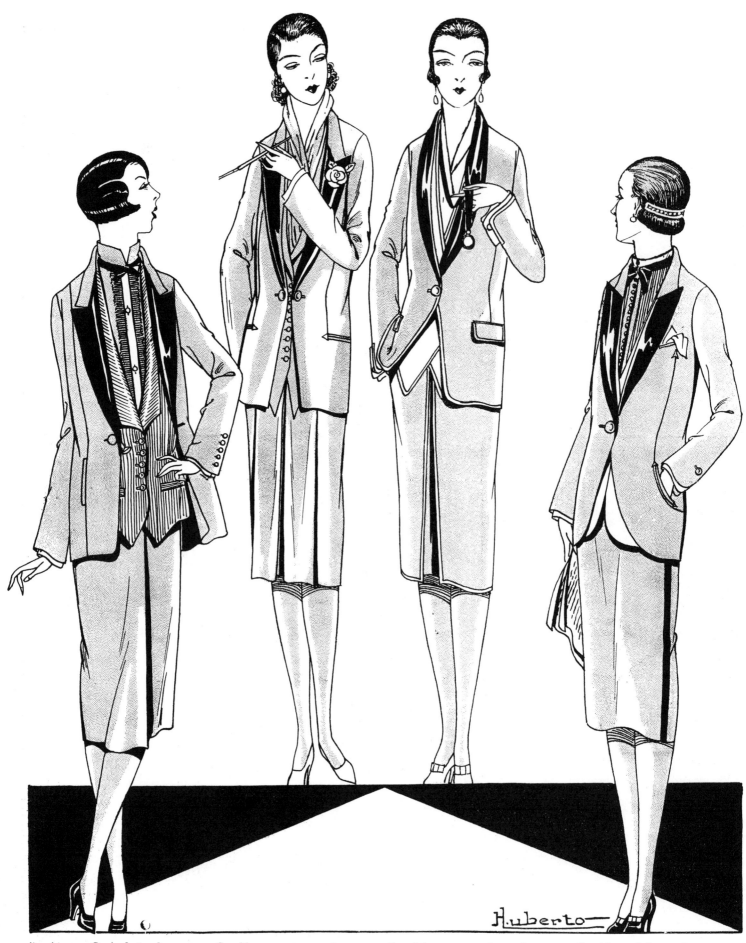

Smoking en Grain de poudre noir, revers de soie, gilet en gros ottoman gris.

Black "grain de poudre" "smoking," silk revers, wide-ribbed grey ottoman waistcoat.

(1264)

Smoking en serge de soie « ivoire ». Gilet de lamé d'or, camélia d'or.

Ivory silk serge "smoking," gold lamé waistcoat, gold camellia.

(1265)

Smoking en reps gris clair ; col châle en satin, gilet en reps de soie blanc.

Light grey rep "smoking," satin shawl collar, white silk rep waistcoat.

(1266)

Smoking en lainage « prune », revers de soie du ton. Gilet de soie crème.

Plum coloured woolen "smoking," matching silk revers, cream silk waistcoat.

(1267)

LES SMOKINGS

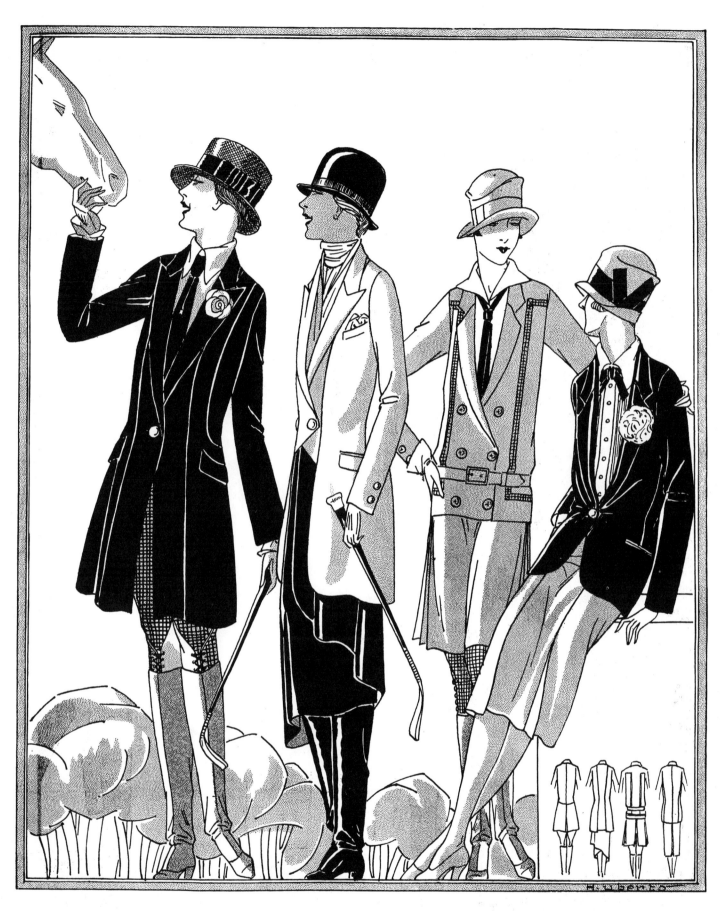

Redingote en draperie marron sur une culotte à damiers marrons et blancs, chemisier de toile de soie blanche; cravate en foulard à pois, bottes beige.

Brown woolen frock-coat over brown and white checkered breeches, white "toile de soie" blouse, tie of dotted foulard, beige boots.

(1716)

Redingote en reps de laine blanc sur une jupe marine relevée sur des bottes acajou.

White woolen rep frock-coat, over navy blue skirt, mahogany coloured boots.

(1717)

Tenue fantaisie en lainage uni et quadrillé, petite jupe fixée à la culotte sur les coutures des côtés, élargie par des plis quadruplés. Chemisier de piqué blanc.

Plain and checkered fancy woolen costume. Short pleated skirt attached to the breeches at the side seams. White piqué blouse.

(1718)

Pour conduire, smoking marron sur une jupe beige rosé. Blouse en crêpe blanc.

Brown smoking over pinkish beige skirt. White crêpe blouse.

(1719)

THE VOGUE FOR HORSEBACK RIDING

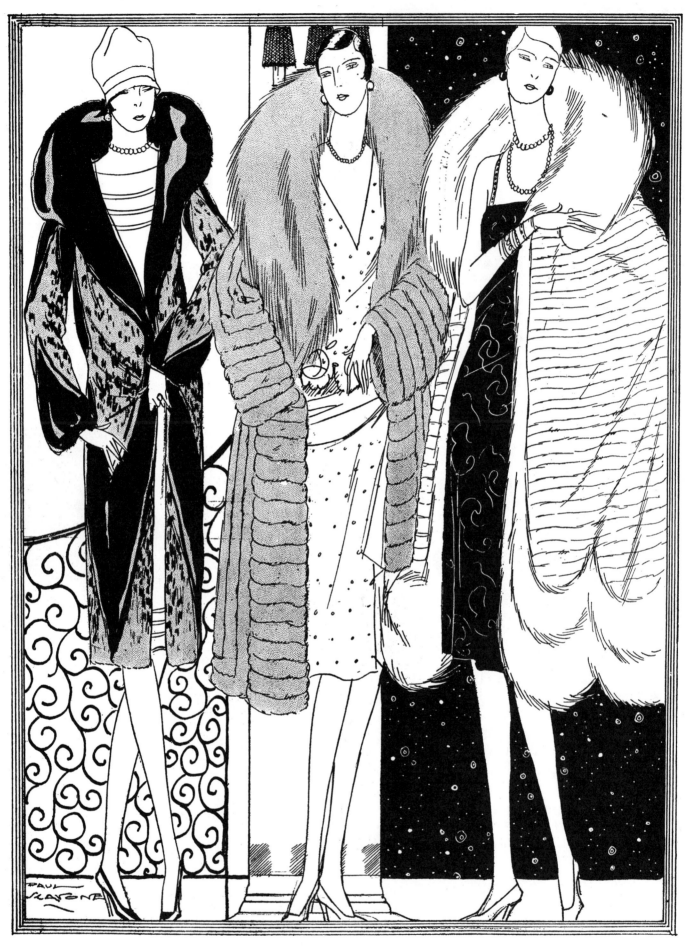

PRÉLUDE. — *Manteau en loutre et veau marin.*

Otter and seal coat.

IMPÉRIAL. — *Manteau en petit gris, col renard platiné.*

Squirrel coat, platinum fox collar.

LINCOL'N. — *Cape en hermine et renard blanc.*

Ermine and white fox cape.

A LA REINE D'ANGLETERRE
249, Rue Saint-Honoré

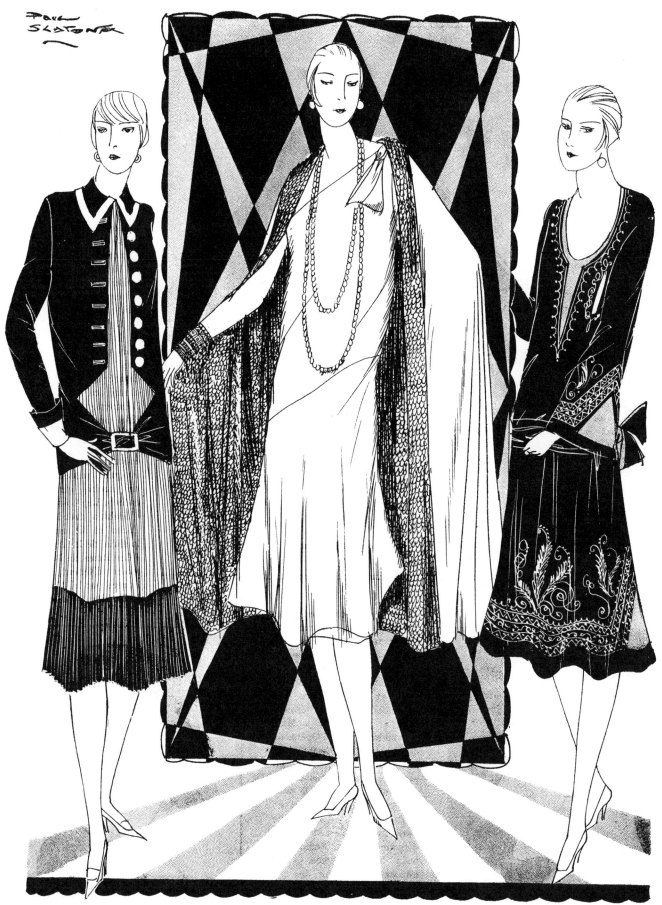

TAMBOURIN. — *Robe de crêpe de Chine noir et blanc.*

Black and white crêpe de Chine gown.

AVALANCHE. — *Robe de crêpe satin blanc, cape en même tissu, doublée de paillettes d'argent.*

White satin crêpe gown, matching cape, lined with silver paillettes.

FAKIR. — *Robe de crêpe de Chine noir et rose brodée d'un ton « ficelle ».*

Black and pink crêpe de Chine gown, embroidered in string colour.

FROM THE NEW COLLECTION OF
NICOLE GROULT
29 Rue d'Anjou.

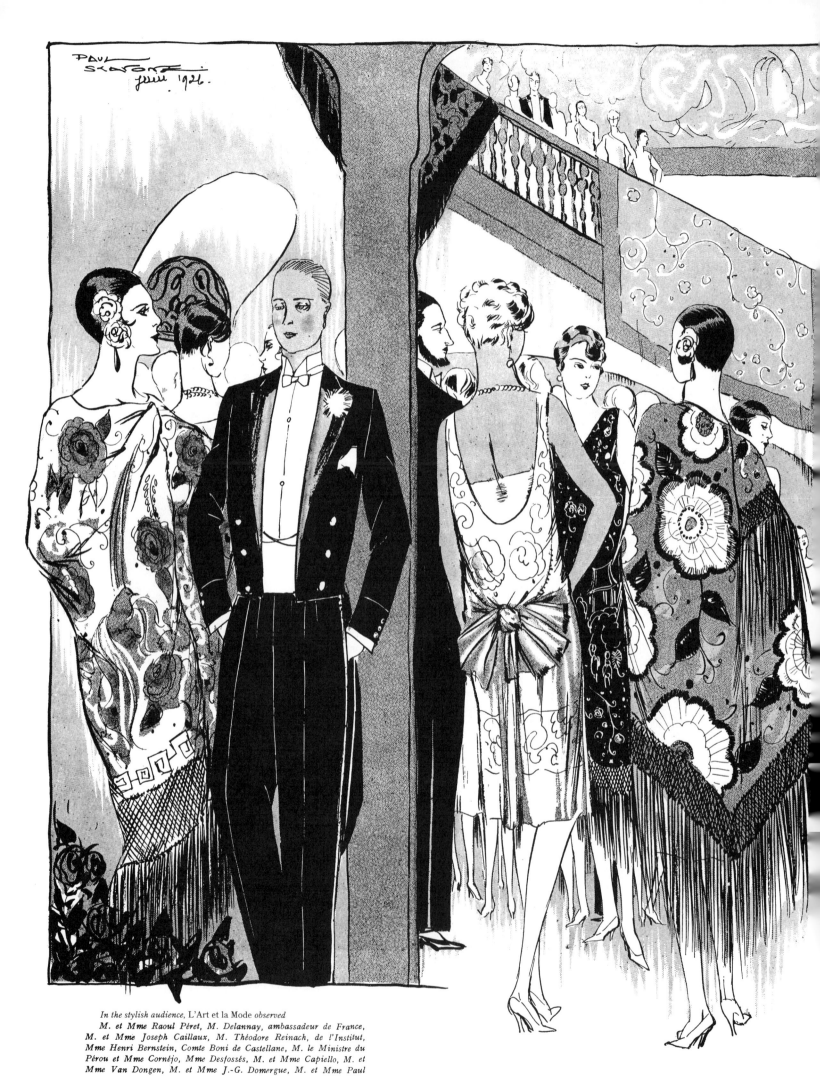

In the stylish audience, L'Art et la Mode *observed*
M. et Mme Raoul Péret, M. Delannay, *ambassadeur de France*,
M. et Mme Joseph Caillaux, M. Théodore Reinach, *de l'Institut*,
Mme Henri Bernstein, Comte Boni de Castellane, M. le Ministre du
Pérou et Mme Cornéjo, Mme Desfossés, M. et Mme Capiello, M. et
Mme Van Dongen, M. et Mme J.-G. Domergue, M. et Mme Paul

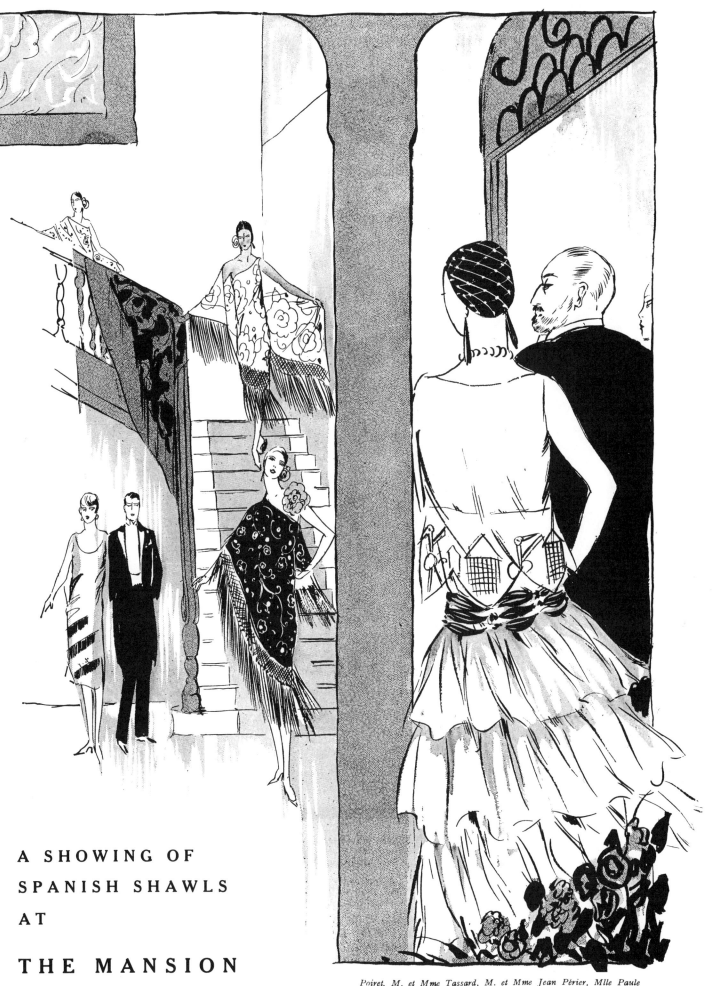

A SHOWING OF
SPANISH SHAWLS
AT

THE MANSION
OF MADAME B...

Poiret, M. et Mme Tassard, M. et Mme Jean Périer, Mlle Paule Andral, M. Romain Coolus, Mme Henri Lapauze, Mlle J. Aghion, Mme Weill-Goudchaux, Mme Benedictus, Mme Bally, Mme Mady Vallière, Mme Féret, comtesse de Crisenoy, Mme Robin, M et Mme J. Darnethal, M. et Mme J. Lartigue, Mlle Régina Camier, M. Pierre Pradier, M. et Mme Balliman, etc., etc.

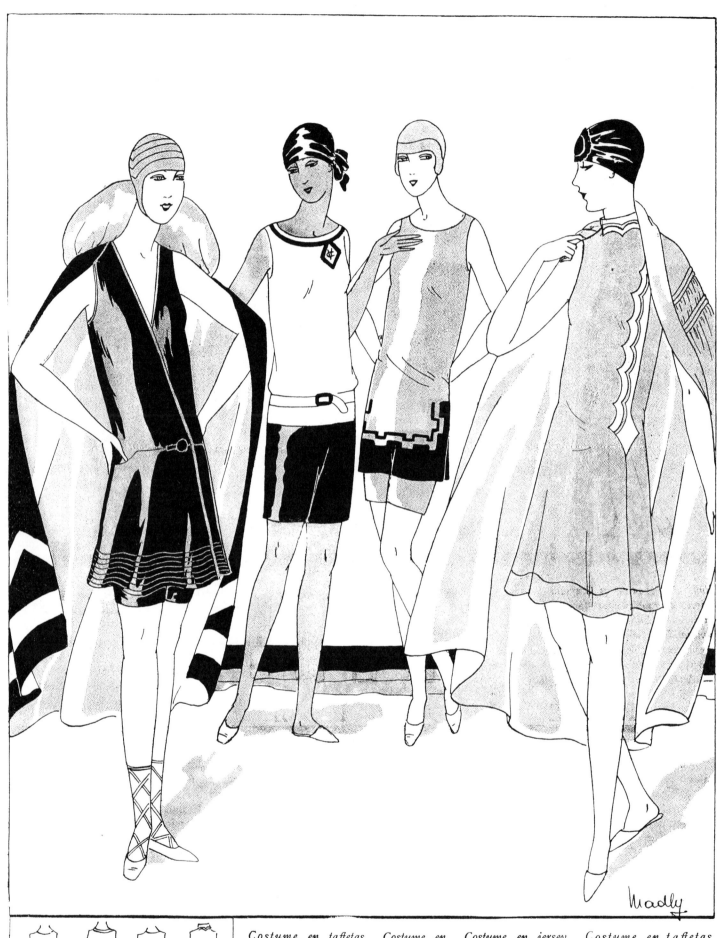

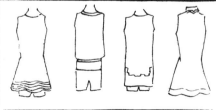

Costume en taffetas marine piqué, cape marine doublée de blanc.

Navy blue taffeta piqué costume, navy blue cape lined in white.

(1703)

Costume en jersey rouge et noir.

Red and black jersey costume.

(1704)

Costume en jersey bleu incrusté de même tissu marine.

Blue jersey costume inset with same fabric in navy blue.

(1705)

Costume en taffetas parme, incrusté de taffetas blanc, cape blanche.

Parma violet taffeta costume inset with white taffeta, white cape.

(1706)

Madly

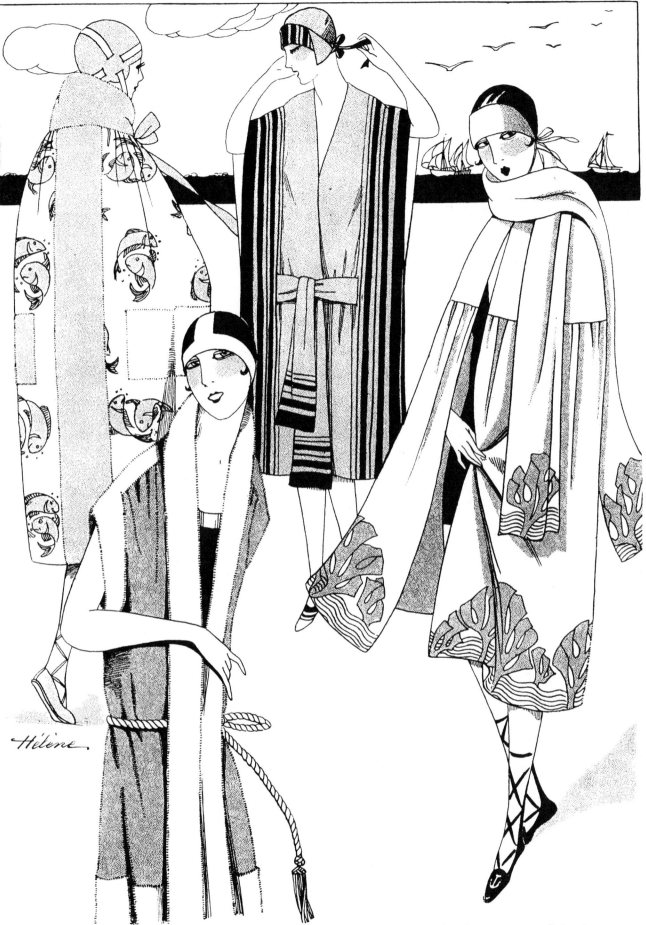

Cape en tissu éponge blanc
à poissons manda-
rine. Bande de tissu
éponge mandarine.

*White terry cloth with mandarin col-
oured fishes. Mandarin coloured terry
cloth bands.*

(1760)

Elégante sortie de bain
en gros lainage « ficelle »,
larges rayures noires,
vertes et jaune d'or.

*String coloured heavy wool
beach robe with black, green
and gold stripes.*

(1761)

Cape en tissu éponge
avec applications
d'algues en tissu
éponge « corail ».

*White terry cloth cape, seaweed
appliqués made of coral terry
cloth.*

(1762)

Peignoir en
tissu éponge
de
deux tons.

*Beach robe of
terry cloth in
two colors.*

(1763)

BEACH ROBES

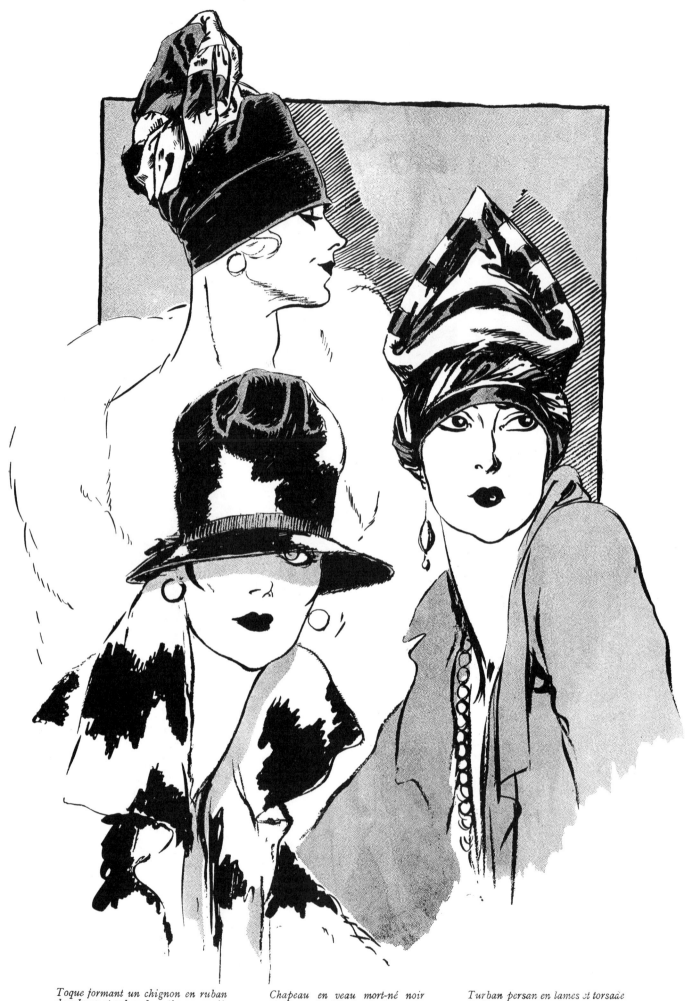

Toque formant un chignon en ruban
de velours et ruban de satin rouge vif.

Bright red satin ribbon
and velvet ribbon « toque ».
MARIA GUY

Chapeau en veau mort-né noir
et blanc, doublé de feutre noir.

Hat of black and white unborn calf, lined
with black felt.
AGNÈS

Turban persan en lames et torsade
de Duvetyne et velours marron.

Persian turban of brown
velvet and Duvetyne.
SUZANNE TALBOT

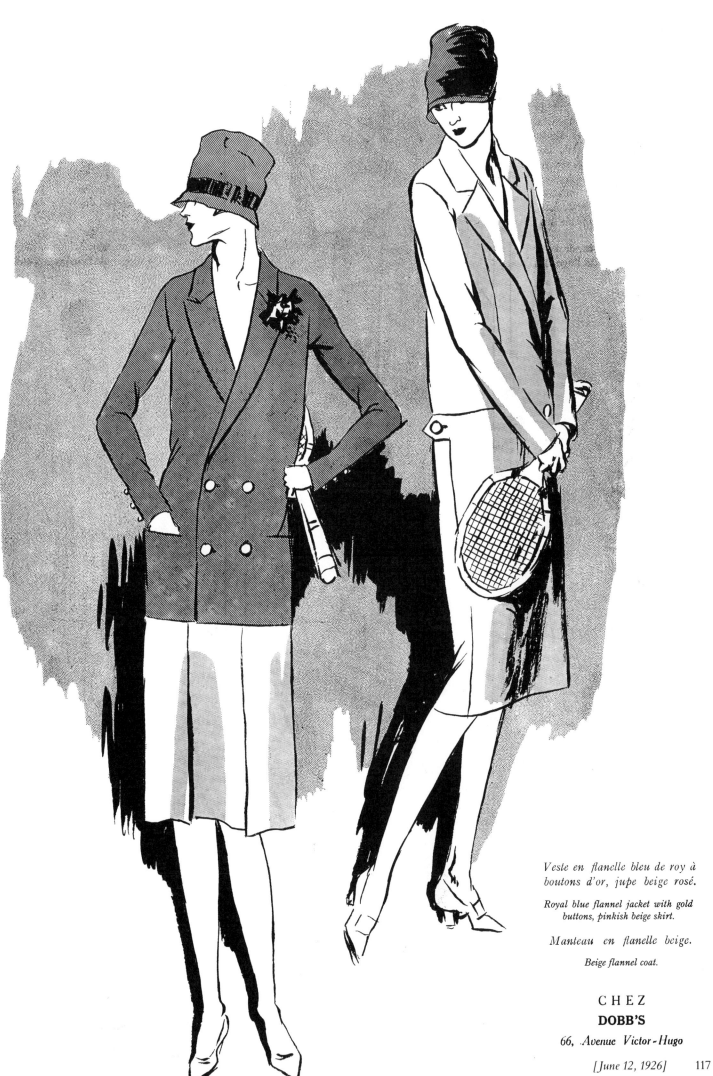

*Veste en flanelle bleu de roy à
boutons d'or, jupe beige rosé.*

Royal blue flannel jacket with gold
buttons, pinkish beige skirt.

Manteau en flanelle beige.

Beige flannel coat.

C H E Z
DOBB'S

66, Avenue Victor-Hugo

[June 12, 1926] 117

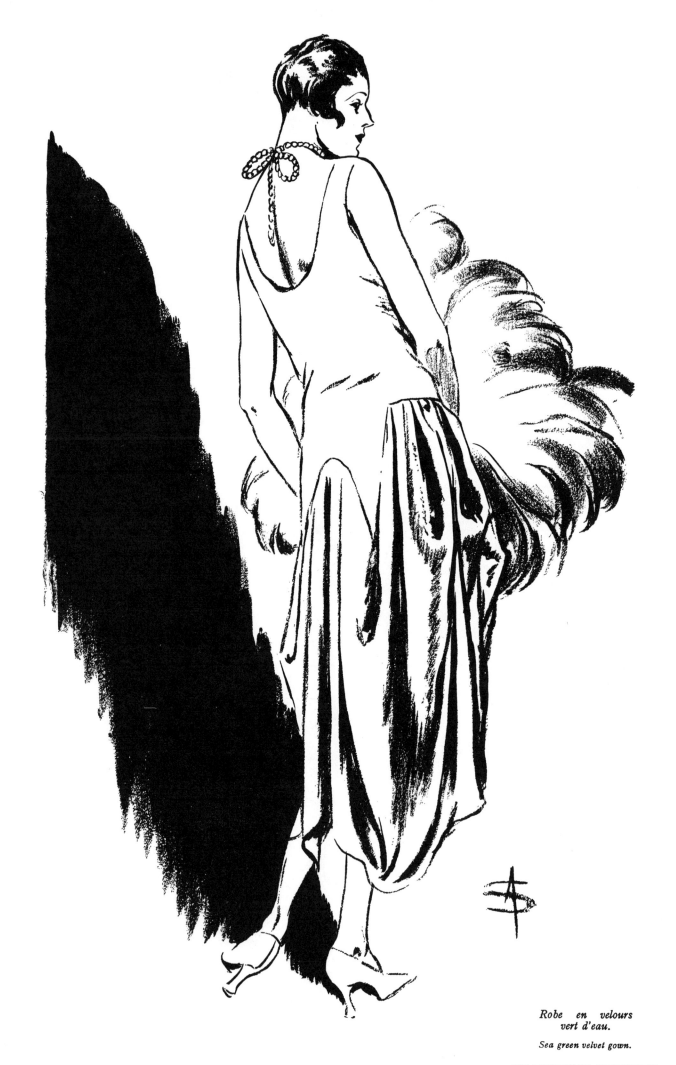

*Robe en velours
vert d'eau.*

Sea green velvet gown.

MADELEINE VIONNET

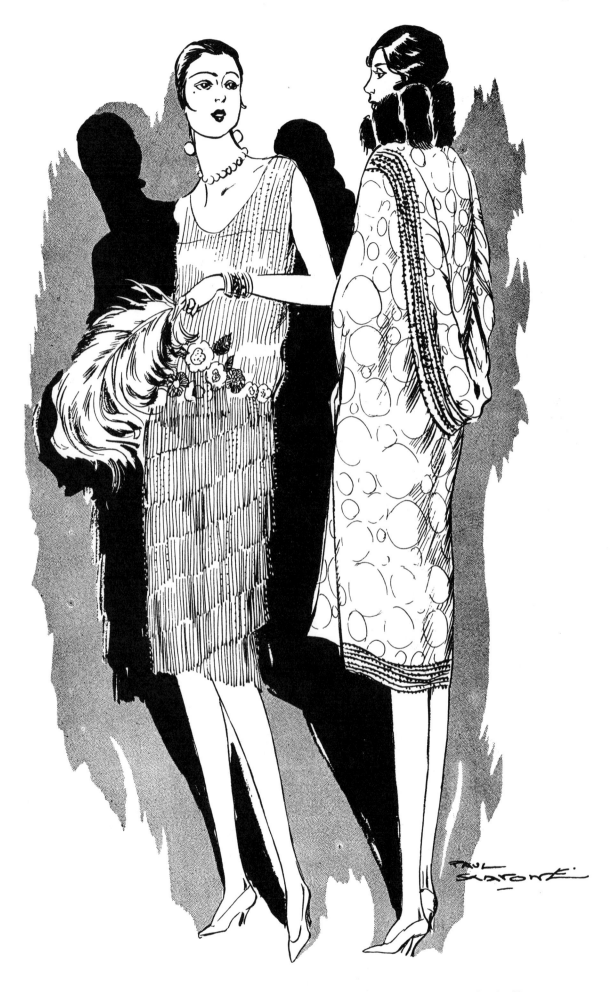

Robe perlée de cristal, blanc,
rose et vert sur un fond rose.

Gown beaded with white, pink
and green crystal over pink slip.

Manteau du soir de lamé multicolore brodé
de perles d'or. Col de petit-gris lustré.

Multicoloured lamé evening coat embroidered with
gold beads. Squirrel collar.

CHEZ GERMAINE
24, Rue Pasquier, 24.

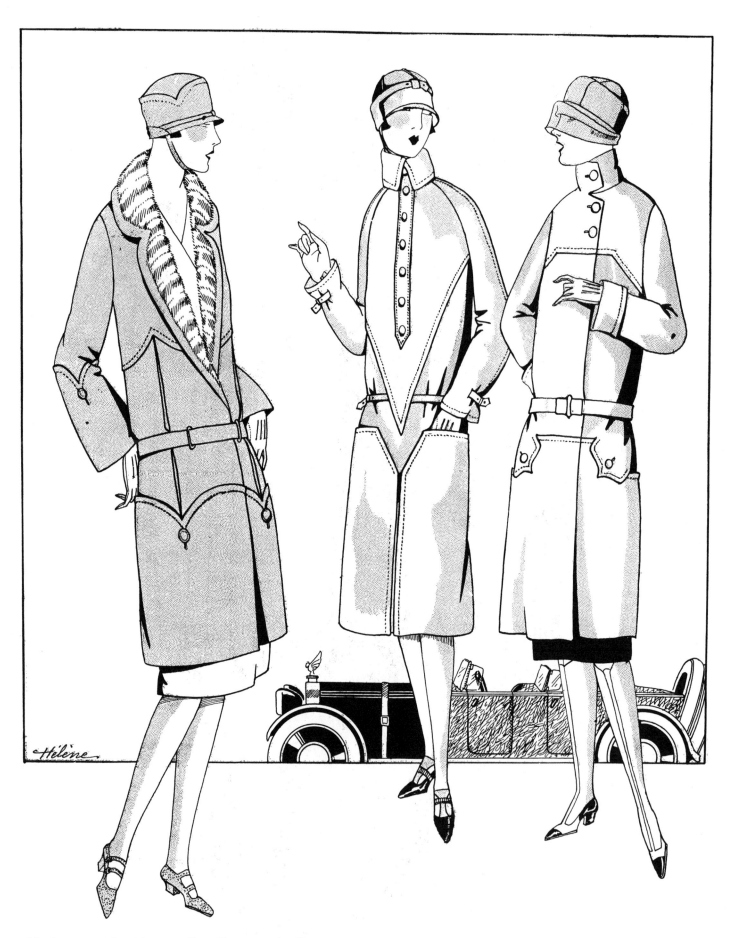

Manteau en cuir violet, grand empiecement et bas de jupe découpés en larges festons piqués, plis creux. Intérieur de petit gris.

Violet leather coat, yoke and lower part scalloped and stitched, box pleats. Siberian squirrel lining.

(1605)

Manteau en cuir fauve, lanières de cuir à la taille et aux manches. Ce manteau s'enfile par la tête, boutonnage au milieu de l'empièement.

Fawn coloured leather coat, leather straps at the waist and sleeves, buttoned to the middle of the yoke.

(1606)

Manteau en cuir blanc, garni de piqûres.

White leather coat, trimmed with **stitching**.

(1607)

LEATHER CAR COATS

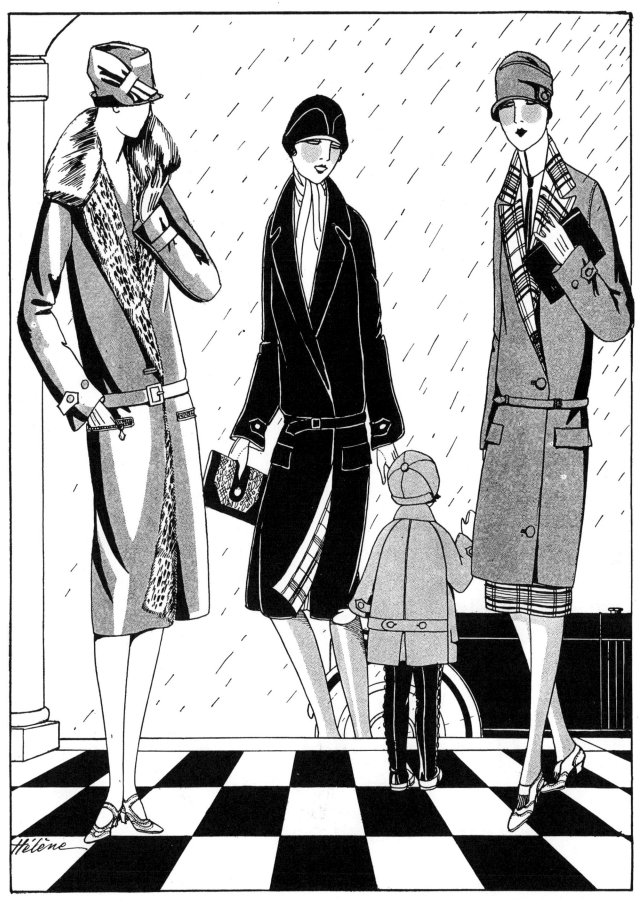

Manteau en cuir « bordeaux » entièrement doublé de susliky avec col en renard, poches à fermeture « éclair ».

Claret coloured leather coat lined with susliky, fox collar, pockets with zipper closings.

Manteau en velours imperméabilisé marron, doublé de taffetas écossais.

Brown waterproof velvet coat, lined with plaid taffeta.

Manteau d'enfant en cachemire beige.

Beige cashmere child's coat.

Manteau en cachemire rouge entièrement doublé de Kasha fantaisie écossais, et jupe en même tissu que la doublure.

Red cashmere coat, lined with plaid Kasha, matching plaid skirt.

THESE COATS ARE INDISPENSABLE FOR RAINY DAYS

CREATIONS BY
LÉDA

5, Rue Drouot

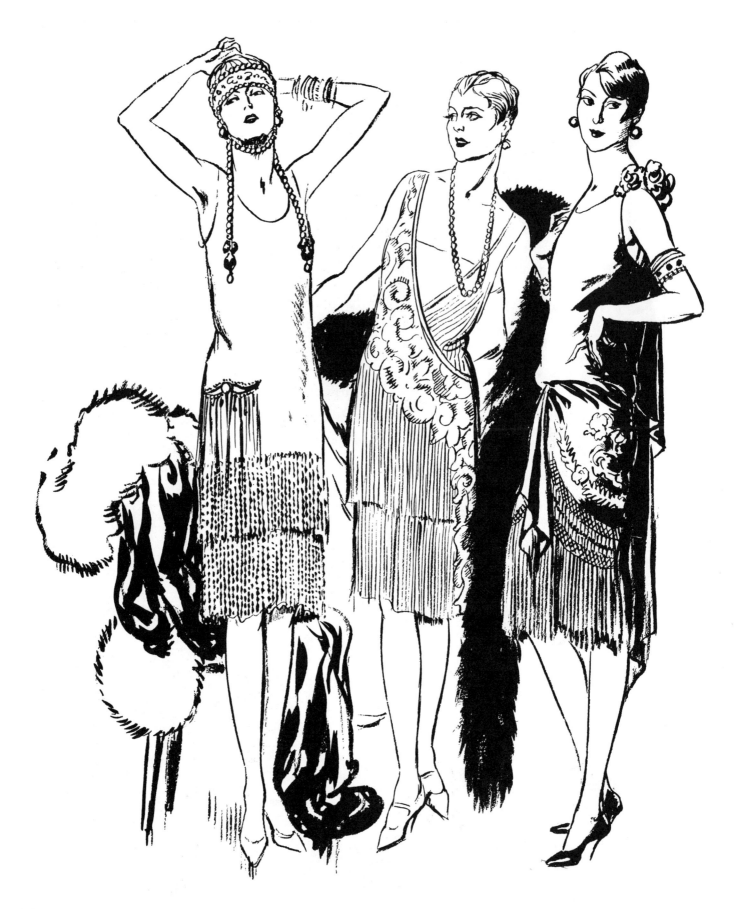

Robe en velours Tircis *rose garnie de franges en laminette argent. Boucle d'argent et de perles fines.*

Pink Tircis velvet gown, trimmed with silver « laminette » fringes, silver and pearl buckle.

PHILIPPE ET GASTON

Robe en pailleté dégradé rose, franges d'argent sur fond rose.

Shaded pink sequined gown, silver fringes over pink slip.

PHILIPPE ET GASTON

Robe en crêpe Romain noir brodé d'or et de différentes couleurs ; franges noires.

Black Roman crêpe gown, embroidered in gold and different colours. Black fringes.

MARTIAL ET ARMAND

CHRISTMAS

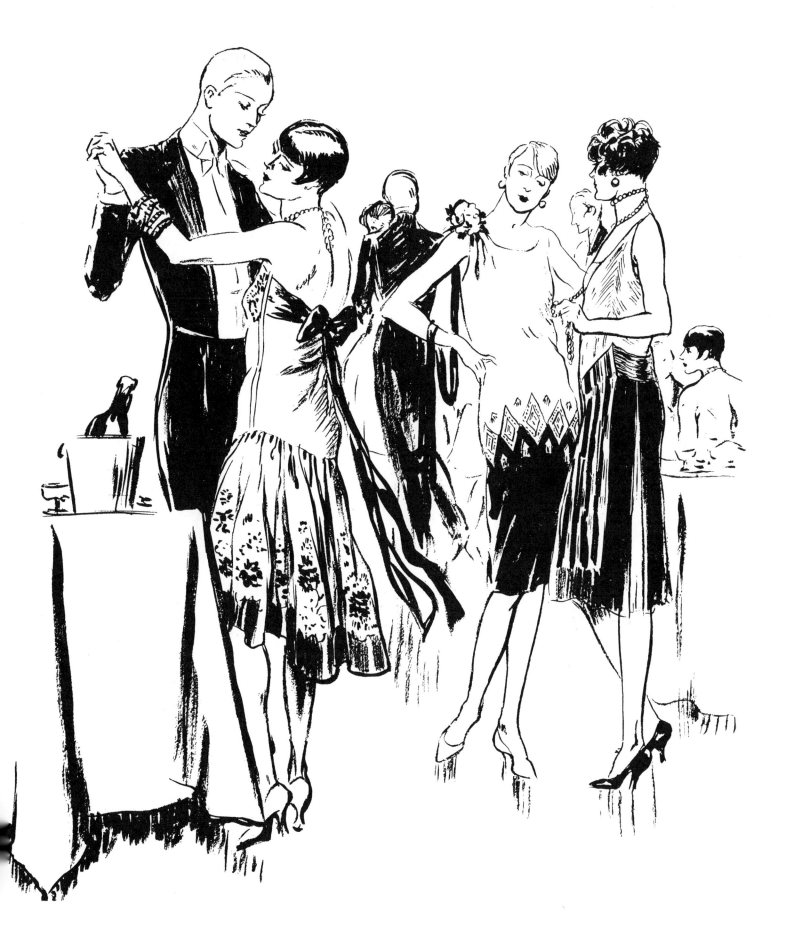

Robe en lamé broché vieux rose, ruban de velours
bleu pastel, jupo garnis de broderies de paillettes d'or.

Gown of lamé brocaded in old rose, pastel blue velvet ribbon,
skirt trimmed with embroidery of gold paillettes.

JENNY

Robe en satin noir et satin
blanc, broderie de strass.

Black and white satin gown,
rhinestone embroidery.

TOLLMANN

Robe en mousseline de soie
noire et rose, broderie d'or.

Black and pink chiffon
gown, gold embroidery.

LUCIEN LELONG

EVE

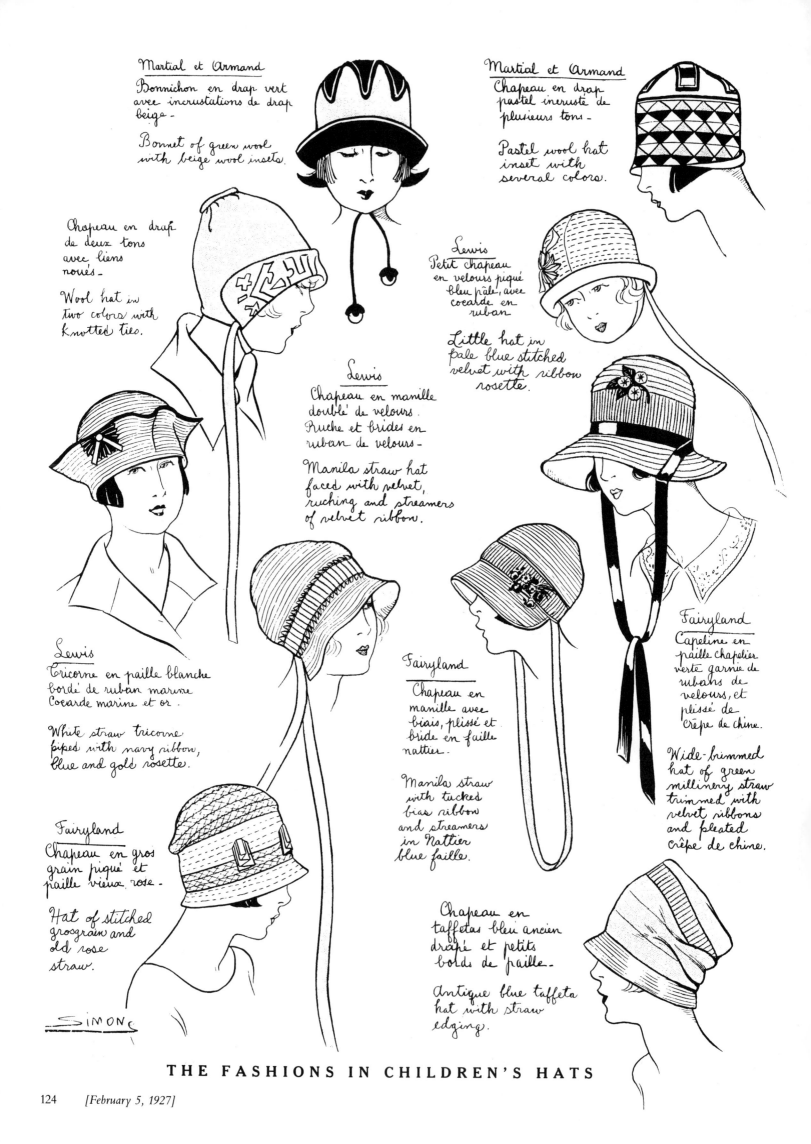

Martial et Armand

Bonnichon en drap vert avec incrustations de drap beige -

Bonnet of green wool with beige wool insets.

Martial et Armand

Chapeau en drap pastel incrusté de plusieurs tons -

Pastel wool hat inset with several colors.

Chapeau en drap de deux tons avec liens noués -

Wool hat in two colors with knotted ties.

Lewis

Petit chapeau en velours piqué bleu pâle, avec cocarde en ruban

Little hat in pale blue stitched velvet with ribbon rosette.

Lewis

Chapeau en manille doublé de velours. Ruche et brides en ruban de velours -

Manila straw hat faced with velvet, ruching and streamers of velvet ribbon.

Lewis

Tricorne en paille blanche bordé de ruban marine Cocarde marine et or -

White straw tricorne piped with navy ribbon, blue and gold rosette.

Fairyland

Chapeau en manille avec biais, plissé et bride en faille nattier -

Manila straw with tucked bias ribbon and streamers in Nattier blue faille.

Fairyland

Capeline en paille chapelier verte garnie de rubans de velours, et plissé de crêpe de chine.

Wide-brimmed hat of green millinery straw trimmed with velvet ribbons and pleated crêpe de chine.

Fairyland

Chapeau en gros grain piqué et paille vieux rose -

Hat of stitched grosgrain and old rose straw.

Chapeau en taffetas bleu ancien drapé et petits bords de paille -

Antique blue taffeta hat with straw edging.

SIMONE

THE FASHIONS IN CHILDREN'S HATS

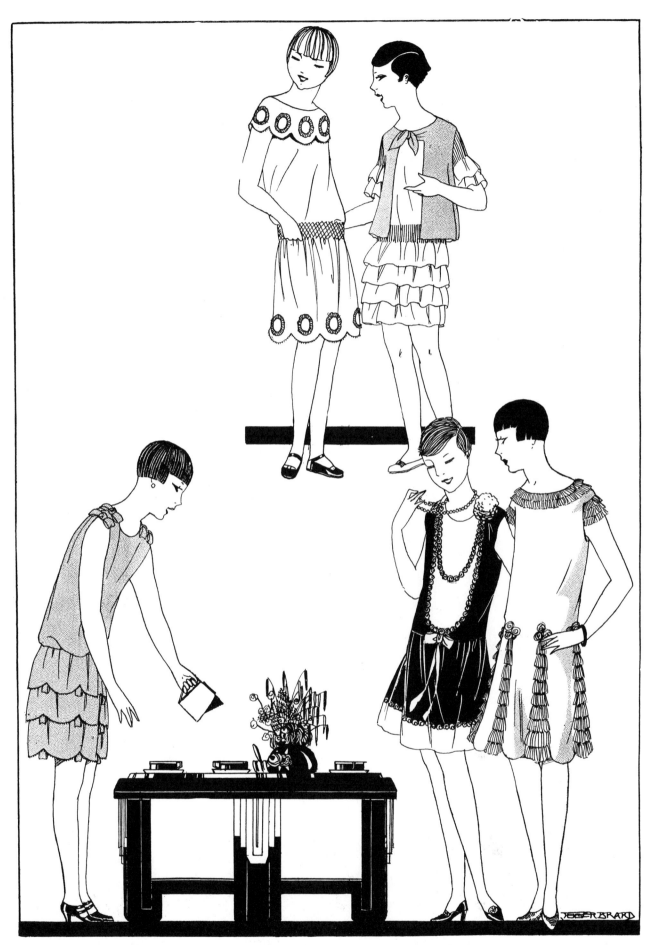

Robe en crêpe « Matou » pêche, garnie de ruban de velours bleu gaufré.

Peach coloured « Matou » crêpe gown, trimmed with blue frilled velvet ribbon.

(766)

Robe en « Organdina », petits plis et volants. Boléro en **velours rose**.

« Organdina » gown, small tucks and flounces, pink velvet boléro.

(767)

Robe en crêpe « Crapote » rose pâle, garnie de rubans de velours du ton.

Pale pink « Crapote » crêpe gown, trimmed with matching velvet ribbon.

(768)

Robe en « Fulgurante » mauve et crêpe « Georgette » blanc, broderie de petites roses roses.

Mauve « Fulgurante » and white « Georgette » gown, small pink embroidered roses.

(769)

Robe en crêpe « Nounette » bleu pâle, petits plissés en même crêpe. Petits bouquets de roses roses.

Pale blue « Nounette » crêpe gown, trimmed with tiny pleats, small bunches of pink roses.

(770)

CHILDREN'S FASHIONS

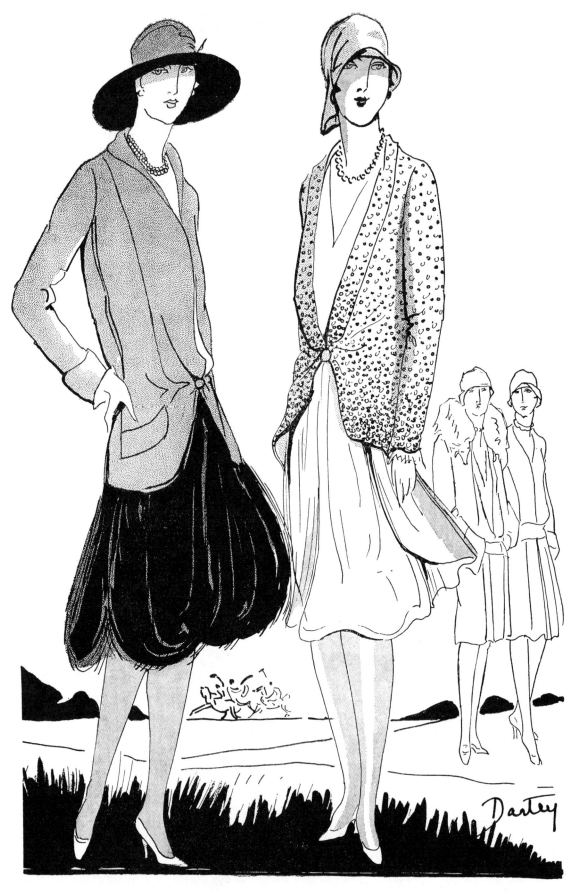

CHÉRUIT   CHÉRUIT

AN EXPRESSION OF STYLE AT "POLO DE BAGATELLE"

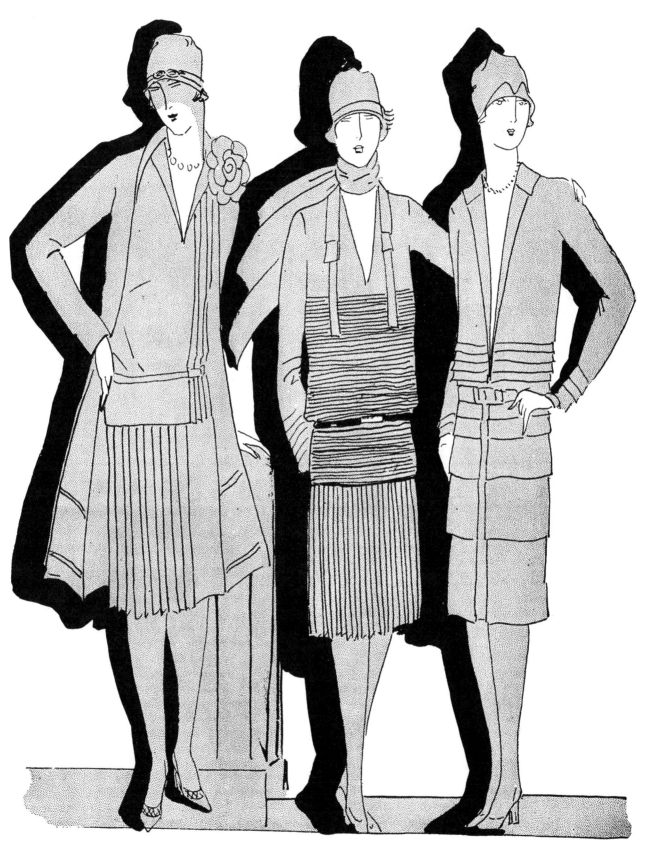

Robe en crêpe de chine bleu
lin. Manteau en lainage bleu.

Flax blue coloured crêpe de chine
dress, blue wool coat.

DRECOLL

Robe en « Kasha »
rose.

Pink « Kasha
dress.

DRECOLL

Robe en crêpe
« Marocain » rouge.

Red «crêpe Marocain»
dress.

MOLYNEUX

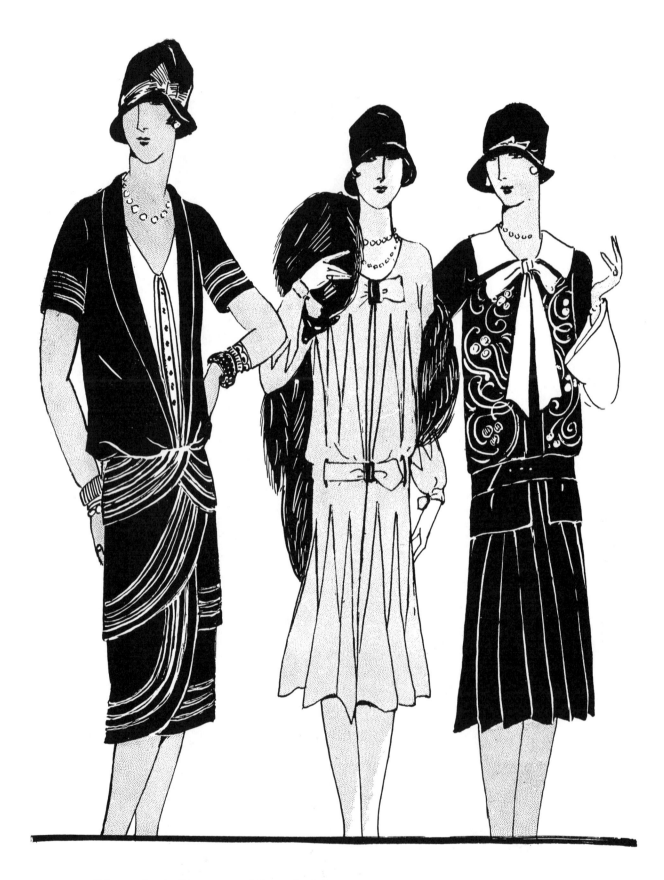

Robe en crêpe de Chine,
garnie de petits biais.

*Crêpe de Chine dress,
trimmed with narrow bias.*

WORTH

Robe en crêpe de Chine
vert amande.

*Almond green coloured
crêpe de Chine dress.*

JEAN PATOU

Robe en crêpe « Marocain » bleu marine
brodée blanc, col-cravate et poignets blancs.

*Navy blue «Marocain» dress, embroidered
in white, white collar, tie and cuffs.*

JEANNE LANVIN

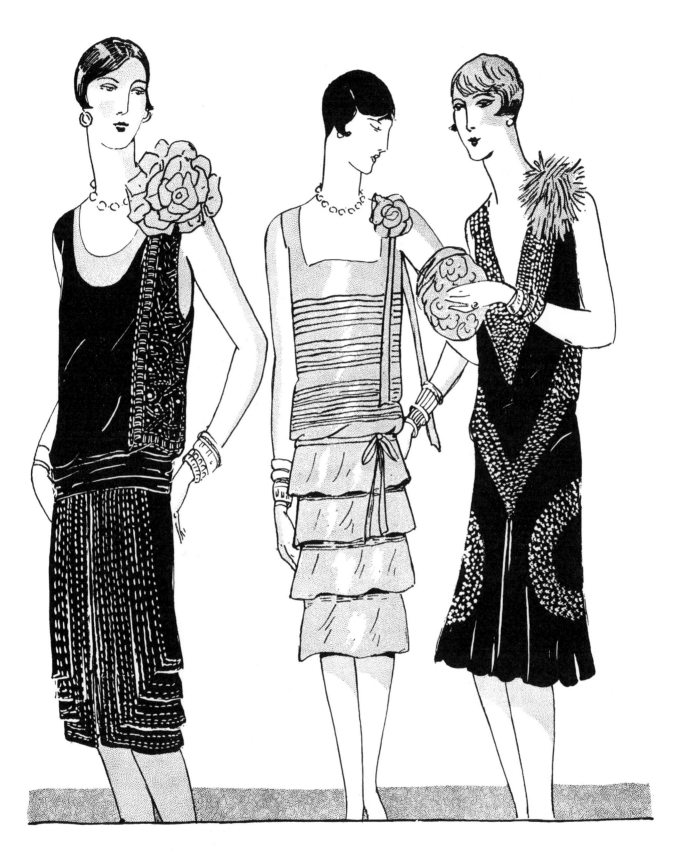

Robe en crêpe « Marocain »
noir, brodé de strass

*Black «crêpe Marocain» gown,
embroidered with rhinestones.*

WORTH

Robe en crêpe de Chine
parme, petits plis.

*Parma violet crêpe de
Chine gown, small tucks*

NICOLE GROULT

Robe en crêpe « Georgette »
noir, brodée de strass.

*Black « Georgette » gown, em-
broidered with rhinestones.*

NICOLE GROULT

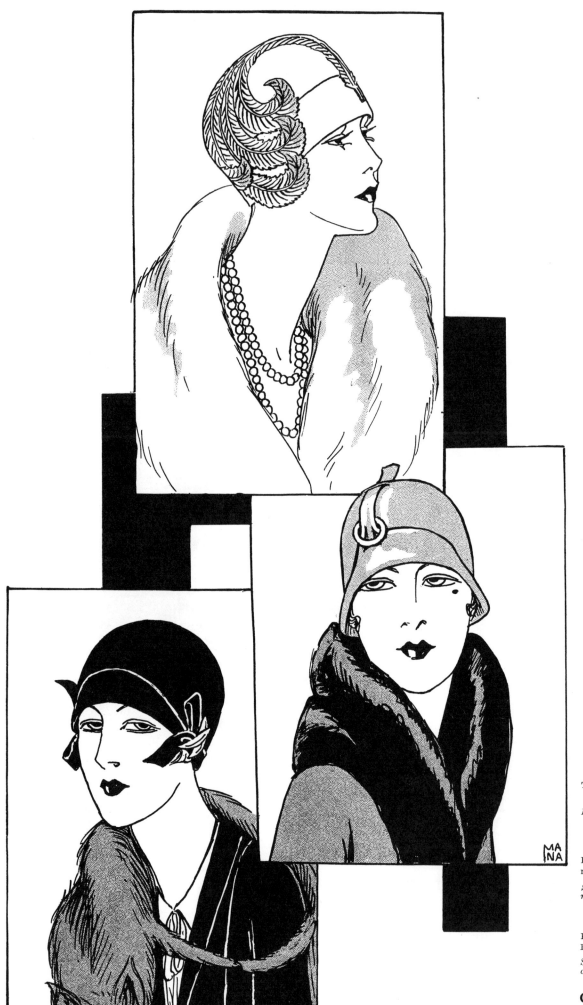

Toque en feutre beige, ornée de plumes pyrogravées.

Beige felt toque, trimmed with pyrographed feathers.

Petit chapeau en feutre noir, orné de motifs d'or.

Small hat of black felt, trimmed with gold ornaments.

Petit chapeau en taupé Bordeaux et anneau d'or.

Small hat of claret coloured fur felt, and gold ring.

CAMILLE ROGER

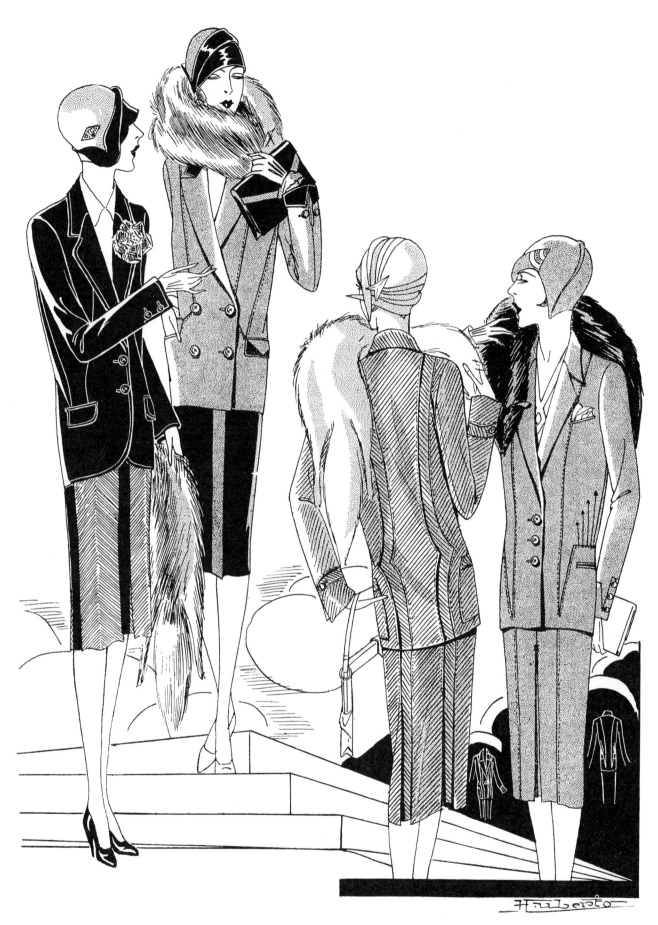

Veste de velours noir, fleur en serpent,
jupe bordée en lainage fantaisie gris beige,
élargie par quatre gros plis. Bande de velours
entre chaque plis.

*Black velvet jacket, with snakeskin flower,
skirt of grey beige fancy wool, trimmed with
four box pleats, velvet band between each
pleat.*

(1509)

Veste de drap beige croisée,
garnie de velours marron. Jupe
portefeuille en velours marron
avec bande de drap beige.

*Double-breasted jacket of beige
cloth, trimmed with brown velvet.
Skirt of brown velvet with beige
cloth.*

(1510)

Tailleur de lainage rayé
blanc et noir. Jupe à
empiècement et plis corres-
pondant aux découpes.

*Suit of woolen material striped in
white and black. Skirt with yoke,
pleats.*

(1511)

Tailleur en tweed gris clair,
pinces en relief sur les côtés
terminées par des mouches. Jupe élargie par un gros pli creux.

*Light grey tweed
suit, skirt with
box pleat.*

(1512)

TAILORED SUITS

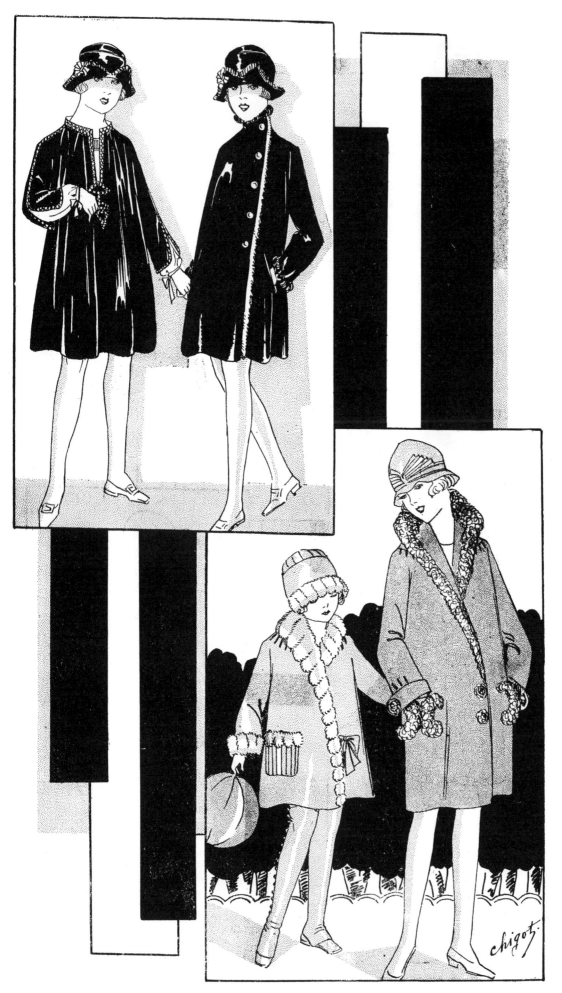

« Infante ». — Robe de velours de soie noir, ornée de grébiches d'argent et de crêpe rose.

Dress of black silk velvet, trimmed with silver nailheads and pink crêpe.

« Werther ». — Manteau de velours de soie noir à godets et fourrure blanche, boutons boules en acier.

Matching coat of black silk velvet with godets, white fur, steel ball buttons.

« Mirliflor ». — Manteau de drap jaune pâle, garni de fourrure taupe dentelée.

Pale yellow cloth coat trimmed with scalloped mole.

« Dagobert ». — Manteau en ratine marine, garni d'astrakan gris.

Navy blue ratiné coat, trimmed with grey astrakhan.

FAIRYLAND

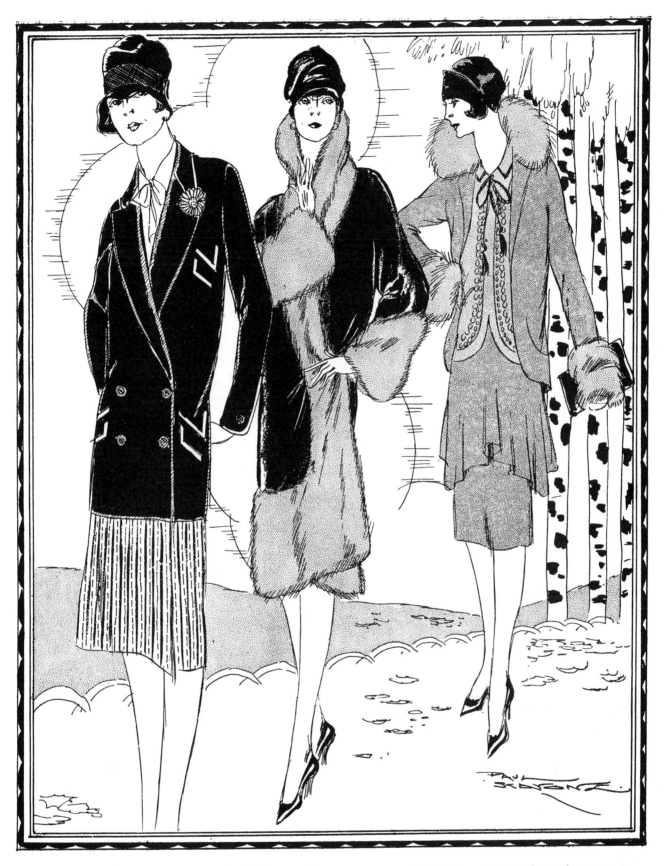

« Falzar ». — Tailleur
en velours noir et jupe
en tissu fantaisie.

*Black velvet tailored
suit with fancy mate-
rial skirt.*

« Les Andelys ». — Man-
teau en lainage rouge,
garni de ragondin.

*Red woolen material
coat, trimmed with
nutria.*

« Jeunesse ». — Robe en velours noir, corsage en
lainage rouge vif brodé de perles d'argent, jaquette
en velours noir, col et parements de renard beige.

*Black velvet dress, bright red woolen bodice, embroidered
with silver beads, black velvet jacket, beige fox collar and
cuffs.*

CHEZ

GEORGES ET JANIN   *25, Rue La Boëtie.*

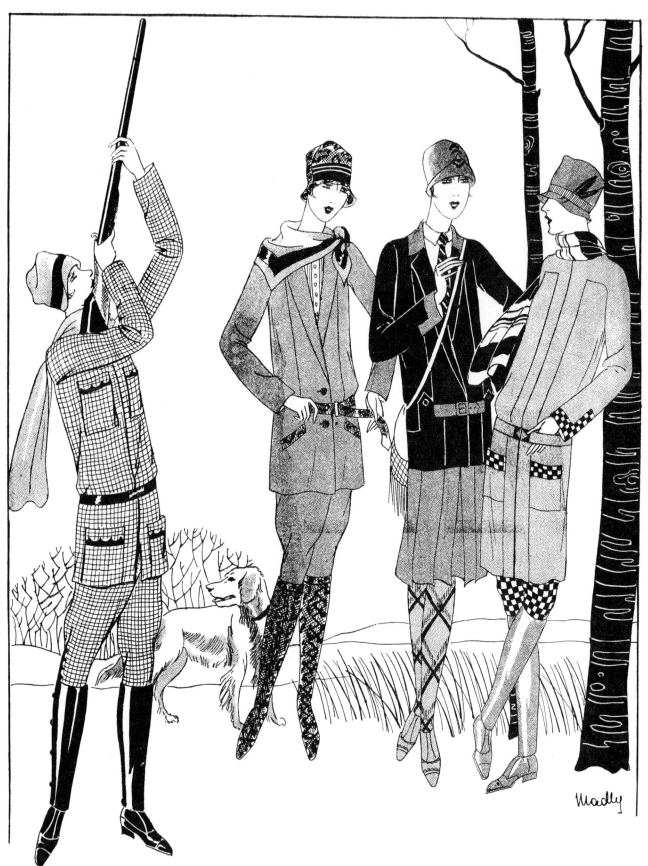

Costume de lainage quadrillé
beige et marron ; bottes et
ceinture de verni marron.

*Beige and brown checkered
wool costume, brown patent
leather boots and belt.*
(917)

Costume en « Kashadrap »
vert bouteille, garni de boa ;
bottes et chapeau en boa.

*Dark green « Kashadrap » cos-
tume, trimmed with boa snake,
boots and hat of boa snake.*
(918)

Costume en velours
cotelé marine et
« Kasha » gris.

*Navy blue ribbed
velvet and grey
« Kasha » costume.*
(919)

Ensemble en serge bleue
et lainage à carreaux
marine et blanc.

*Blue serge and navy blue
and white checkered wool
ensemble.*
(920)

THE HUNTING SEASON OPENS SOON

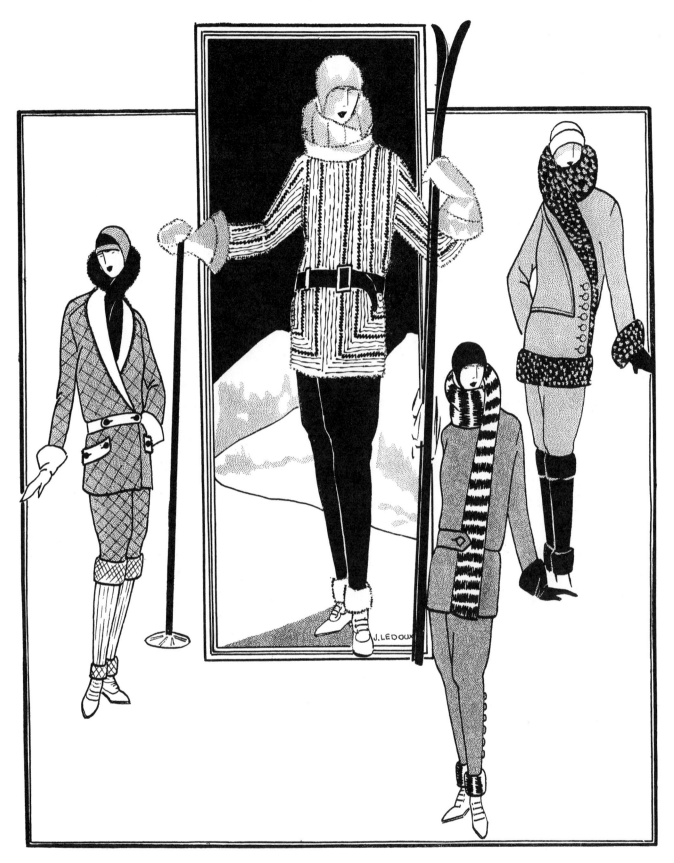

Costume de sport en « Diaburavelline », garni de piqûres formant quadrillé. Parementure de tissu blanc uni. Chandail de laine rouge.

Sport costume of « Diaburavelline », trimmed with stitching forming squares. Plain white lapels. Red wool sweater.

(1582)

Costume de sport en Angora blanc et rouge ; col de lapin blanc, culotte de tissu imperméabilisé rouge.

White and red Angora sport costume, white rabbit collar, red waterproofed trousers.

(1583)

Costume en tissu imperméabilisé vert clair, garni d'un grand col écharpe de laine pékinée noir et blanc.

Light green waterproofed costume, trimmed with large scarf collar of black and white stripped wool.

(1584)

Costume en Angora bleu, boutonné de côté et garni de fourrure de laine pointillée.

Blue Angora costume buttoned on side, trimmed with spotted wool.

(1585)

FOR WINTER SPORTS

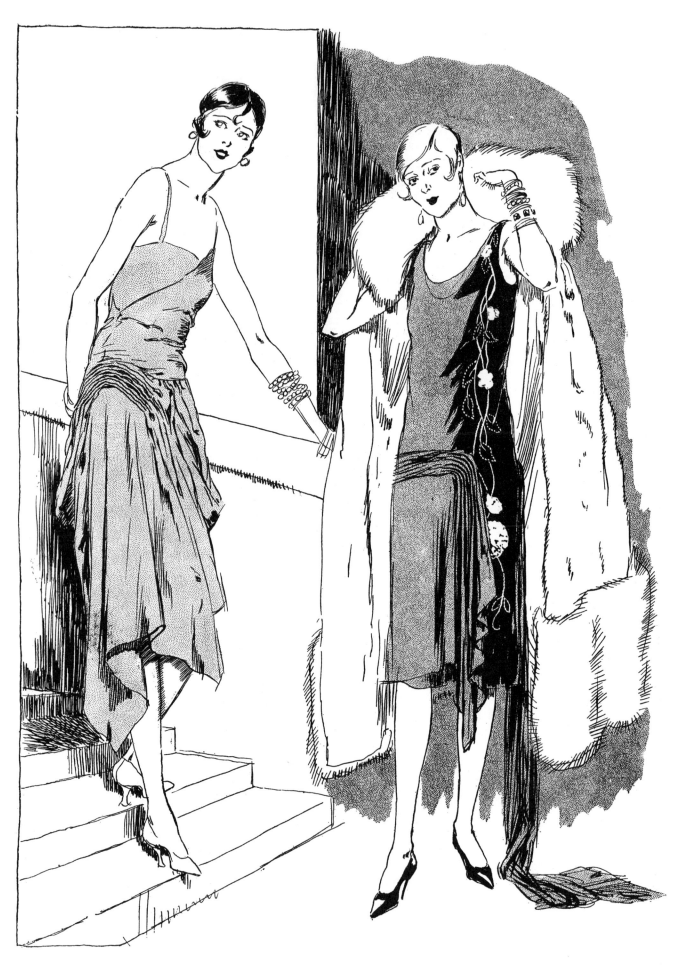

Robe de dîner en
satin Duchesse rose.

Pink Duchesse
satin *gown.*

MOLYNEUX

Robe de dîner en « Georgette »
noir, brodée de gardénias blancs.

Black « Georgette » gown, em-
broidered with white gardenias.

MOLYNEUX

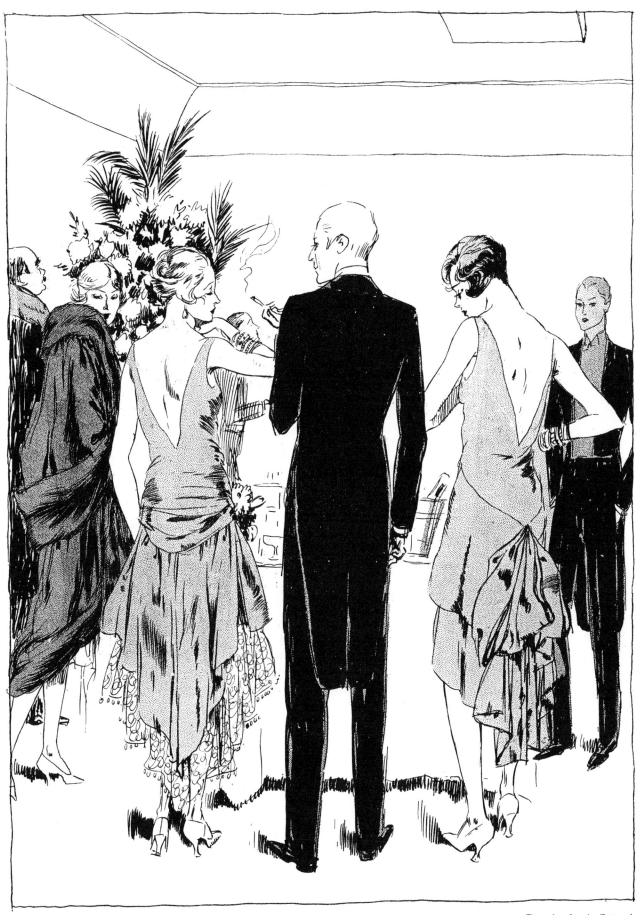

Drawing by A. SOULIÉ.

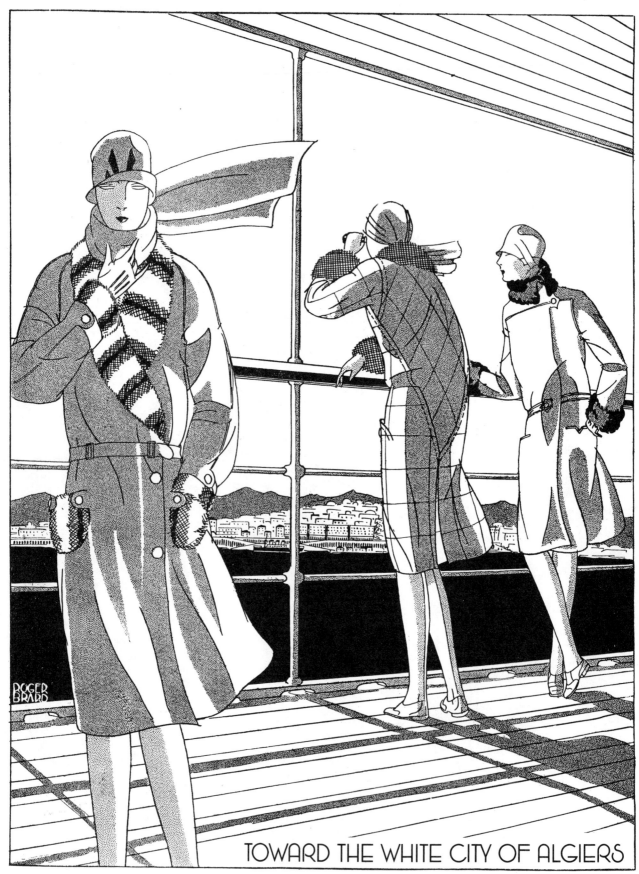

TOWARD THE WHITE CITY OF ALGIERS

Manteau en « Kasha » doublé de ventre
de petit-gris et garni d'oppossum.

*Coat of « Kasha » lined with squirrel
and trimmed with opossum*

(1648)

Manteau en gros lainage quadrillé
ton sur ton ; parements de fourrure.

*Coat of heavy checkered
woolen material, fur cuffs.*

(1649)

Manteau en peau chamoisée,
col et poignets de fourrure.

*Coat of chamois leather, fur collar
and cuffs.*

(1650)

THE MEDITERRANEAN CRUISE